How Not to Die

Overcoming the Incurable: Hope, Love and Resilience - An Inspirational Guide for Patients and Families.

Nathan Delfim

This is a work of fiction. Names, characters, places and incidents are either the product of the author's imagination or are used fictitiously, and any resemblance to real people, living or dead, business establishments, events or places is entirely by coincidence.

Dedication

The short story is dedicated to those suffering from incurable illnesses. All those suffering from incurable diseases and their families who give up their own lives to be near their loved one, and to all the people who only have eyes to look at the skies in hope or to find an answer.

Moms who hide their feelings, who cry quietly and secretly. They have to practice smiling in the mirror once they come out from that place. Mothers who are never tired and who win every battle. Mothers who are always in the background, who can't describe their pain when losing a child.

All mothers, those who have given birth, raised children and led their lives, please light up!

For those who don't feel hot or cold to secure the future of their heirs. When the separation feeling from your children is strong, you cannot stop them. They are the ones who have rough hands and old shoes. Or the one's with the identical suit hanging on the rack. They are the ones who never stop searching for salvation to save their children.

The fathers who have a sick child want to be woken up!

The book is dedicated for all caregivers, wherever they may be. People who choose to be caregivers as their profession. Patients are identified by white shirts and the angel wings in their eyes.

Preface

Sophia died at an early age. She became a role model for those lucky enough to have met her even once. Her smile, which was filled with light, was unique, as was her movement.

She was greeted by everyone with a smile, like a star shining in the sky, whenever she passed the city. It wasn't just her external beauty, but also the light she radiated and spread everywhere that attracted people to her.

Sophia was fighting the illness for quite some time and this separated us from her. Sophia's incurable illness was a shock to all who knew her. It came at a time when it had reached a very advanced stage, and she could no longer fight the disease. Today, I still hear friends repeat the same phrase:

She managed to maintain all of this weight by herself.

Sophia probably had the hope of one day succeeding and telling everyone about her life and how she did it.

"It's too cold outside for me and I lean on the window railing every morning to be inspired by the music. It's pouring rain. The window allows me to see all the living and not-breathing things.

Even the rain seems to have frozen my emotions. Sophia thought, "I feel the warmth from the cup of coffee in my hand."

I always stop my gaze at a large tree, which is not able to withstand the rain drops. It looks as if it's suffering. The wind is causing it to sway from side to side, and it shows no mercy to its leaves and branches. When I see it, I find myself right there!

From the window it appears that the tree is older than 20 years. It seems to me that the tree has existed for a long time before I opened my window. I have never paid attention to its suffering or beauty.

The seasons have changed. I can't believe that 20 years have gone by. From my window, I can see that it still stands, but it is suffering from its shape and wounds on the trunk.

This tree is strong, adaptable, and seems to be indestructible. It has never fallen.

Sophia - I'm curious now! What can I do to find out the age of this tree from? I thought to myself.

I was disturbed by the sounds and my mind became a mess. The TV was off and I leaned back against the window. I was very interested in every little detail! What is going to happen today with this tree? What can I learn from this tree?

The tree is so old, strong and big. It doesn't seem to be aged at all. There are marks of pain on every inch of the tree, but this makes it more beautiful.

The old man ran towards the tree. He was dressed well but had no protection. It was obvious that he didn't foresee these downpours. His only weapon was his stick, which helped him make two legs.

He might have gone for a stroll, I thought. The unexpected rain made it difficult for him to walk. It looks like the stick is part of him, and it speeds up his steps. From a distance, I can see that he wanted to get shelter and was walking towards the tree. It was exactly what happened. His body language made it clear that he felt safe and protected under the tree.

It was frightening at times to see the wind bringing rain into my home. While holding my breath I put the cup of coffee on the table in the living room and ran to the man. He was sheltered by the branches of the wonderful tree. I saw him thanking the tree with his eyes. But that wasn't enough, I had to offer him somewhere warmer.

The life cycle of the tree dominated my mind as I hurriedly went down the steps. "Majestic! This tree has a mission that is not only to resist temperature changes and weather variability but also to protect!" I said to myself.

How many people did it shelter in all those years? Who knows how it can make them feel safer? The old man may have known this tree and walked until he found it. They were definitely friends. This tree must have given this man a great deal. Perhaps it even protected him on hot days. They are definitely friends.

He raises his eyebrows often. Sometimes he smiles. I've seen him talk to the tree. They've probably been good friends for years! I was thinking of approaching him.

Please, come with me home, as you're not safe. It is freezing and raining. Come with me into my apartment and warm up. "I will then accompany you home." He said.

Michael: "Dear lady, I thank you for your concern but feel secure here." He said

Sophia: Please, Mr., if you don't come with me home, you are in danger. I spoke to him in a firm voice as though I knew him well.

After a brief moment of reflection, he smiled and began to walk towards me.

When I grabbed his arm, I thought I was helping him to walk. But I actually felt more protected by him. We both got wet on the way up to the gate.

It didn't affect us negatively, and it seemed to calm my spirit when the rain fell heavily on me. Even though the cloth was wet, I felt it as soon as it touched my face.

Sophia: You were right. I feel just as safe in this rain. "I said, smiling.

He smiled and then we laughed until we were inside my apartment. My feelings have gotten warmer and I am sure that one day, too, I'll find refuge under the same tree. "I said it to myself." I knew this tree would give me something very special.

Michael: Lady, the room is freezing cold. You should do something to warm it up! He suddenly said.

Sophia: I'm sorry, mister. I can raise the thermostat now, if that is what you prefer, even if it is only 22 degrees in there. Then I'll prepare some hot soup and hope that it will stop raining so I can accompany you back home. You are welcome to stay with me. - He answered me in a timid voice.

Michael – What's your name, lady? - He told me that the sentence was not intended for that purpose.

Sophia: My name is Sophia. For everyone, it's Sophia. Strangely, my father calls me Eli. You, sir? What is your name?" - I asked him smiling.

Michael: You are a beautiful person, Sophia. Michael is my name, and I'm 74. I don't mean to talk about temperature in degrees but rather about the warmth of your soul. The house looks very neat, with everything in place. This is only noticeable when there's loneliness. He said it without hesitation and without considering that we didn't know each other.

Sophia: Mister Michael you have the same beautiful name as me and I am delighted to be able to meet you. He laughed in an emaciated voice. The room was silent and I needed to do something to end it.

Sophia, I'll make you some hot tea right now. I broke that silence.

Michael: Thank you. I'd drink that with great pleasure. He smiled at me when he answered.

To get rid of the strange feeling, I quickly prepared tea. I felt that he knew my entire world. What made this man think I was lonely? It's not true! Perhaps yes? What should I do? This is embarrassing! While preparing tea, I thought and wondered.

Michael: Don't be embarrassed. You know, maybe we won't see each other ever again. My health is up and down right now. I am very sick. I have lived my life believing that everything happens with a purpose. He spoke to me like he could read my mind.

Sophia, you are special! No one had ever offered me hot tea or soup before today, and I've been waiting for it since years! It's not expensive, and I understand that, but I appreciate the gesture. Being polite is free! Under that tree, I've sheltered several times. It has even provided the cooling that is so important in these hot weather conditions.

Sophia: "I understood it. I know it. You've known me for years." Michael - I was proud that I also had managed to grasp something.

Michael: Dear Sophia... Fill this house with harmony, because that is our mission in life... Do not make the mistake I made...! He talked to me while stroking the top of my hair.

We were so lost in our conversation that we did not realize the weather had changed and it was much clearer.

Michael: I must go.

Sophia: If you like, Michael I'll accompany you home.

I actually didn't wish him to go, but I did want to hear his wise words. I asked him for advice. His life experience taught me a lot about myself. Michael said very few words, so it was hard to remember all of his words.

Sophia: Michael, you were a delight to meet, and I thank you so much for your beautiful words. They will stay with me forever! I said it as if this was my last chance to see him. It seemed to me that the way to his home was very short. I did not want to meet him, or to leave him. I knew he was telling me the truth. He said he'd spent all his life like me. Alone!

Michael: Remember these words Sophia. We are what we leave behind. It was his last words to me on the road to his home.

Sophia: Thank you Michael. I look forward to seeing you soon, and to talking under the beautiful tree. We laughed and greeted each other as we parted.

Was ready to begin the day, but was running late. Now that it is too late to have another coffee, I can't. I was leaving for work.

Routine makes people sick. I stop to enjoy, and take in everything around me. Today, I'd rather not drink coffee and have a good feeling. I thought.

... Michael' last sentence was not very clear to me. What did he really mean?

The meaning of "We are what we leave behind us" was something I had to repeat to myself many times.

One day, I'll find out what this sentence means. I told myself that it was time to forget about this sentence.

It was so beautiful, big, strong... I couldn't stop looking at it. The tree was beautiful, big and strong. It was always admired for its bravery. The wounds in its trunk were so beautiful because it had been through every possible weather problem. It was for this reason that I gave it a unique name to match its circle of life.

Life is what I call it!

It's a damn shame, but I just can't take this cigarette! - When I was a teenager, I wasn't thinking about smoking. I dislike being around smokers. It's not my fault that I smoke.

The smog in the city is not a joke, but it's affecting our health day-by-day.

Oh, yes I am aware... I criticised myself loudly.

You need to get up, my love. Today you'll also be fighting with your customer. I was encouraged and went to work like every day.

Aaron: "Good morning Sophia. As always, you are on time."

Every morning, it's the same: the same words, the exact same expression, the exact same eyes. It is true that he's one of my co-workers, but it would be more accurate to say I'm his boss. I don't like being called a colleague. He does it every day, with a big smile on my face, and achieves the goal.

It seems to be an anti-stressor for him. He gets more done, and it sometimes gives him hope. Especially when I say Good Morning, Dear. But since today wasn't a day for hope, he was satisfied with a simple smile.

Aaron was working for us since a year and I even selected him to be on the staff. He's too polite and is an excellent orator. His dialectic is unmatched. He is an economist, but I often think of him as a talented and dedicated journalist.

I was aware that I wasn't just his colleague, or even his chief. I needed to maintain his productivity and I gave him a small sign to finish his day.

It was even possible that, one day, if I had to start a family I might have to keep it from him. I was worried that he'd leave. But the truth was that I couldn't work without him. He was indispensable. In truth, I had to admit that deep inside I wanted to keep something from myself.

How can my personal life be so intertwined with my work life? It would be wonderful to live a normal, happy life like the two people I saw from my office window)....

Aaron was talking, and I saw it on his face.

Aaron: Sophia, I'm sure today is not the best day. It's not the best day. I'm sure you are always busy but I can see you from the other side of the glass. You always have your back to the computer in the office. I know how hard you work and that today is a very important day for both you and us, as we await the biggest customer. He said.

He kept talking. It was like he talked to himself. His face was confused, and he couldn't find the words. Because I didn't know what he was saying, I stopped him.

Sophia, Aaron. What's the matter with you? I don't understand you. Take a deep breath and calm yourself down. Then start again. "Smile at me," I replied. My elbows were on the table, and I looked directly into his eyes with both hands. Aaron stared at my hands, then sat in silence. He couldn't speak anymore, I realized.

I felt a strange sensation in my chest! When I wanted him to stop talking, I would always act in this way. I was very aware of how I could stop him, or get him to do what I asked.

Sophia-Aaron, I'd like to talk with you another time. As you have said, this isn't the right day. Perhaps tomorrow.

Aaron - Sophia, tomorrow? I'm too late to react tomorrow, the days pass and turn into weeks and months. I am not that way, I would react in time in the exact same circumstance but under different circumstances. His answer was accompanied by a look of disappointment.

Sophia: Aaron, as you admit, these situations are different. I may have also reacted differently in a similar situation, but under a different circumstance. Let's discuss this at a later date. I replied with a loud voice.

Aaron: What are you trying to say, Sophia? He looked at me with doubt.

Sophia: Maybe I wouldn't have even accepted you coming to my office. Or I would accept but with an agenda! I replied to him, my heart beating hard. I was worried that he would hear it too.

Aaron began to speak, but was interrupted by the office telephone ringing! The CEO was there. It was the CEO.

Aaron had the guts to walk into my office. It wouldn't be long. This situation has come up so many times that I have tried to avoid it. "I repeated it myself."

He was distracted when I looked through the glass of my office. I really needed him today!

What do I need to do? It was important to me that I find a way out.

I was told to tell him a lie by my mind! Even though I considered writing him to say that I'd meet him after work privately, he knew the truth! I thought he was too intelligent to accept that. It would have taken a lot of effort from me, but the important thing is that he wouldn't be able to.

It never occurred to me that I would play with his emotions just so I could achieve my career goals. It made me wonder if my concern for his feelings was really about mine. I was motivated to solve the problem as soon as possible after seeing him unmotivated.

Coffee would have made the situation worse, so I ordered tea. The tea was the most likely choice. The best choice was probably tea.

After this, I am sure he'll be better today. I'm proud of the choice that I made. Aaron's unpredictable nature was not something I considered. He could mess with my emotions, and give me the direction he desired. He had to have been able to handle those two tea cups and still surprise me.

Aaron took the cups, but there was no sign of my tea. I assumed he had been so mad at me, he wouldn't bring it to me, but I didn't get up from my chair.

As I watched, he went back to his desk and took out a pen. He then left. But I did not move.

Was worried, had to confess! My whole body was so heavy, and I knew it wouldn't work. But I did not lose hope. I was determined to try something new. I needed to get his attention more than ever.

When I lifted my head, behold!

Aaron was holding a cup in his right hand as he approached my office. While Aaron entered my office, I was feeling proud and repeated it to myself in my mind:

Sophia is always right. This time it worked too!

His smile grew brighter as he approached the office.

Aaron was beautiful, intelligent, gentle and kind... I always enjoyed his company. Every time I saw him, I couldn't control the smile I got.

His intellect was irresistible. A lot of times, I wondered if his intelligence was the reason why I felt so attracted to him.

It was very important for me to be around him in some way.

Aaron: Thank you my dear. That's exactly what I was hoping to discuss. Aaron - Thank you, my dear. That's what I wanted to talk about.

The sentence made me feel relieved. I even closed my eyes in a brief moment of joy. I had no idea what the speaker meant.

His smile made me happy. He sat at his desk with a lot of energy. I saw this from my glass wall.

The tea was not something I wanted to consume. I was busy. Aaron seemed to be working with a lot of concentration and was relaxed. I was tempted to rush in and throw my tea on the floor because of the vase of fresh flowers that was sitting at the corner.

Then I poured it into the pot and stood up, then turned around to see if AAaron was there. It seemed that he hadn't seen anything.

The glass partition was almost broken by the stare of AAaron as I sat at my desk.

He smiled and I placed the cup on the plate. The cup of tea was placed on a plate and he smiled.

It was a bit of a shock to see - on top of the tea cup was tucked t he plate t he paper, folded into four. I knew it had something written in it, and I was afraid of opening it.

Aaron and I looked at each other, but there was a glass wall between us.

Aaron forced me, in a indirect, but persistent way, to read the letter as soon as he realized I'd seen it. He put his pen down, left his computer, and placed both his hands on the desk.

With that look, it seemed as though he were saying something to me.

If you don't read the document, then say goodbye to your customer.

The situation was so confusing that I had no idea what to do. The letter contained what I had been trying to avoid. I read it and I realized that I would have to deal with something new, that which was in my mind but that I did not want to release.

Aaron did not move, he appeared frozen at the same place. It seemed as though everything was prohibited, as if there were no other people, just me, Aaron, the letter and his eyes on me.

Aaron bowed to me and told me I had done the right thing. He made me realize that I needed to open the letter by moving his hands.

After a brief moment, I considered that it would be better to open it and not read it. Instead, I decided to smile at him so he knew I'd read the letter.

I thought to myself: 'What if this letter has nothing that makes me smile?', I pondered. I felt compelled to open it. It was a letter. I looked at it quickly and at Aaron.

Sophia, I am in need of you. Trees need oxygen for life. Aaron!

It was a sad day! It was clear to me. Aaron was not in sight! Why was this happening to me? I had too many thoughts going through my mind! The heartbeat was fast and I was trembling all over. I also started to cry, perhaps as a way of releasing the intense emotional feeling I felt at that time. At the same I felt happy, but also sad. My thoughts were a mystery to me. My thoughts were racing and so was my heart. Closed my eyes, I tried to return to normal. This was not possible!

Aaron was walking towards my office, looking worried.

Aaron: Sophia, I'm sorry, but this wasn't my intent! He put his hands on my palms and said: "This was not my intention!"

He tried to tell me the reason for his actions, while standing on his desk and placing his hands there. Sometimes he would cover his face in concern with a hand when he couldn't speak.

He appeared to be very concerned. He seemed to have lost his only chance of achieving what he wanted.

Aaron: Sophia, forgive me. I did not want to have this happen. But I could no longer handle the feeling! He breathed deeply and said, "I'm sorry."

He sat down and took the chair in front of my face. Without speaking or moving, we just stared at each other. We both seemed to have the same wish, that this moment would never end. The hands on the clock were the only thing that caught his eye. He reached for the tea cup with his left hand without saying a word.

He was about to toss the letter out when I quickly grabbed his arm. I grabbed the letter in my hand and handed it to him.

Both of us laughed when I acted instinctively.

Sophia: Now, promise me you'll do the best job possible today and that everything else will just be forgotten. - He said.

Aaron: I will make sure that you get what you desire, but today's events will never be forgotten. - When he answered, he got up and grabbed my chin using his fingers.

Aaron was able to keep his promise. It seemed like he forgot everything. I thought that I'd seen a nightmare. Everything looked so normal.

His reaction to the client was reassuring.

All went as expected.

I was required to attend dinner meetings with clients, but after what happened with Aaron, I thought about the best way not to appear at the meeting. My feelings were a mess and I wanted to reflect alone.

At that point, it was as though I were reading his mind. He imagined that I would be wearing a completely different outfit to what he is used to, and sitting with three other people at a table. But he only wanted my company. This would never happen. Aaron was not going to have a good day today, even though I had no control over the situation.

Aaron was the one who saved me from the unbearable pain. I thanked him for his help and complimented him for the day.

Sophia: Aaron, I'm not feeling well. You will be accompanying the client tonight without me.

Aaron did not seem to be at all concerned by my rejection. He even thanked for the compliments he did not deserve. I was leaving work in secret and didn't tell anyone goodbye.

When I got home, i called my CEO to tell him about the extension of contract for three more years. He was told all of the details. Aaron would take my place, I said.

Henry: "Sophia I have no doubts. Thank you. "May I ask why you went home so early?" He was very concerned.

Sophia: "I'm not feeling well, I have high fever, but I am going to try and get better soon." I said as if there was no need to be concerned.

Aaron's Letter was still in the pocket of my jacket. I grabbed it, leaned up against my window and read and reread it. It's hard to say how many times I have read the letter. Aaron's words reminded me of my life tree.

It was just to let me know that he needs me. Maybe he felt the same way as a tree in the rain, and he wanted to stop that rain from falling.

What is so special about me? What will become of both us now?

It is not tomorrow that I am going to work, but it will be all other days. It is important to say that I don't see any hope in this situation, as I could not imagine it.

I thought and tried to convince myself nothing had happened, that it would all be back the way it was very soon. It was so strange that I couldn't understand it. After saying goodbye to my Life tree, I left the window. Even the book that I was reading, which was about letting feelings go free, was a focus of mine. I have had those feelings in me so long, but never allowed them to come out. The disappointments in the past made me take even more extreme decisions.

From my window, I saw the tree Life smiling at me. It was as if it embraced me with its branches and sheltered from afar... My tree, Life, smiled back at me through my window. It was as though it had embraced and protected me far away with its branches. Every day, it made me feel like a good friend and yet I found time to visit. It's possible I was scared that if she met me, I would feel emotions I had already denied myself. I had a relaxing day, but not in the way that was healthy. It was important for me to get over what Aaron did yesterday. It was clear that one day would not be enough.

The phone was ringing constantly, but I wasn't expecting any call.

I said, "Sophia, it's time to get back to work." As I walked towards the telephone. Looking up, I saw who had called me. My eyes couldn't take what they saw! I had to rub them twice.

Aaron called me on my personal phone! It was the first time he had done so. Even if the question was about my work, I chose not to respond. He's good at it and can handle everything by himself - that was what I told him out loud

The ringing finally stopped. It seemed to last a lifetime.

Then I exhaled all I could. You exhale so much that it makes you want to exhale all the tension in this moment!

This situation became more challenging for me every day!

It will ruin my life, I have no time to do this. The phone rang again and this time, it was an email. Aaron was the same as yesterday, so I did not want to open it. Aaron wasn't in my presence, and I was not obliged to open it.

Hello Sophia,

Your presence was needed, as I did not know much about the subjects that were raised by the client. I would have benefited greatly from your presence. You aren't at work, and this makes me feel bad. My mission is over now that you have a contract extension for three more years.

You will surely find someone more competent than I. Soon you will realize that there is no such thing as an irreplaceable employee.

"I'm not saying goodbye" because we never know what the future holds. Maybe, one day, we may meet again.

Aaron

Aaron, I've never felt so bad in my entire life! After reading the email, I thought loudly to myself. Unconsciously, tears began to flow from my eyes and I was paralyzed.

Why Aaron ...? Aaron, why?

Eight months ago, I tried to prevent what was happening. Although I knew that he was going to leave, I still needed him at work. Just now, when he's got the job under control. It was so hard to keep him away from work. I cried! This is impossible! I said to myself. It's impossible!

Even I did not want to tell myself the truth. Perhaps the tears flow because I'll miss his constant remarks. Maybe I have gotten used seeing him and thought of how his departure would go? It's true, not only am I thinking of Aaron but I'm also crying.

Sophia: "No, No, It Can't Be True!" I Said Out Loud.

After a moment, I remembered the penalty of his contract and decided to write i>to him/i> as the only way I knew how. I'd already given up my feelings. I also couldn't express the truth. After a brief moment of reflection, I decided that the best way to tell him the truth was to send .

Dear Aaron,

You are appreciated for the dedication and time that you've given to our company. You are free to go, but you must remember that there's a penalty for such leaves. I have signed it.

You cannot replace the role that you are currently covering in one day. You will need to remain in the role for six months before your replacement has been trained.

Thanks, Sophia.

Even after I sent him the email, I was aware that my actions had worsened the situation. The real reason I wanted him to remain was something I could not accept. The truth is, I was never able to get another, but I always thought I would. My phone kept interrupting my thoughts. Aaron called, and I answered, confident that everything was in my hands.

Sophia asked me, "Hello Sophia. How are you doing?" in an extremely persuasive voice. You could not respond to him very easily.

"I have had better days, but I will be back to shape very soon," was my response.

The man laughed and said, "From your e-mail it appears that you're in great shape."

On the other end of the line, I understood my email was meant to convince him to remain.

Sophia: I fully understand the message of your email, but we need to both understand that six months are too long for me. "It's crazy for us both that you don't get it, so let's speed up the process for our sakes." He stated firmly.

You can't just leave. "You cannot leave that way." I calmly said.

I ended the call by wishing him success in his future studies and a positive review for tomorrow. I was well aware of his firmness. I was afraid he wouldn't really show up tomorrow for work. While I was aware of the reasons why I asked him to remain in my presence, I also knew that I didn't want him to leave. The phone rang again, but it had a message. I was so eager to see the message that the phone dropped from my hand.

Aaron had sent a text message. Okay Sophia, I'll be working tomorrow! He wrote.

My strength was gone. Or rather, it seemed as though I had given up on something I couldn't overcome. I couldn't get my thoughts to leave me. How did I escape? I found it difficult to change. When I considered changing myself, I would think of different events that had transformed me. One such event was when I turned seven.

My mother always shakes my hand when we walk in the city. I recall having a doll with me. My curly hair meant I preferred dolls that had straight hair. My mother was stroking my face with her gaze the entire time. She stopped suddenly to greet a woman who doesn't arouse any sympathy in me. As if asking for shelter and strength, I hugged my mother. The lady asked me after greeting and talking with them for a couple of minutes.

What is your beautiful name? She asked. My mother was looking at me, so I pulled my hand and looked hopeful. She's Sophia. Thanks for your compliments. But she is a bit shy around strangers." Mom, who was only distracted for a second, asked what the newspaper she bought every day after we walked together. This lady took advantage and came up to me very closely. She spoke words I will never forget.

The woman said to me, "Beautiful Girls don't Live Long!" in a very low voice. She then left and greeted mom like nothing happened.

This statement made me cry many times. It was the beginning of my life, and it is also how I began to distance myself from others. The only thing I could think of was that nobody ever took the time to really understand me. I fell asleep in a few seconds, tired and weeping, with my thoughts jumbled up. The next morning, I was emotionally exhausted.

Michael came into my mind as I looked at the furniture in the salon. Michael is right! This house is cold. The phone that I dropped before falling asleep was still on the floor. The phone fell from my hands as I was falling asleep. Aaron left his office less than 30 mins ago. But my phone was still unanswered since I last sent him a message. It was a very sad feeling, and I did not want to say that I'd miss Aaron. This non-answer made me think of the eight months I spent in his office. 'Maybe, I did too much?' I wondered.

I picked up the phone to write him. Because I feared I'd make an even bigger mistake, I threw away the note I started writing and put the phone on the ground. Aaron was very important to me, and I didn't ever want him to leave.

I feel a strange sensation in my chest that transforms into non-stop tears. Why was I drowning in tears? "Why did I drown in tears?"

The melody of the music on my glass captured my attention. Rain was falling. It was raining. Life, the tree I love most in my life came to mind. It might help me out of the situation I was in, which I didn't want to be in. So I got off of my sofa and went up front. As the rain fell, it seemed to caress leaves and transform them into water. "How wonderful nature is!" I thought to myself, smiling.

We should also behave in this way. It's not like things just happen. Maybe I should turn my difficulties into strength. You, Dear Life. Then I turned back to the couch and smiled at him. Before I got back on the couch, my eyes were fixed on the phone. I was about to sit down and grab the handset when I turned around. A light foot push sends me under the couch. Leave me alone now! I called you Aaron.

It was a fact that I did not want to acknowledge the war I had with myself. This struggle divided my feelings from logic. I had been guided by logic in the past and felt comfortable. But the other side of the battle was so powerful that it didn't leave me feeling comfortable all day. It was something I cannot describe. This feeling has been talked about and described a great deal.

Even though I thought that I had tried it. It was compared to heartache when no one knew if it hurt or not. Even the phrase "butterflies in your stomach" is often used. The world's most famous poets are sick of this feeling.

How many examples, descriptions and writings can you provide? It was not how I felt. This was not what I felt! The feeling starts with the speed at which the blood circulates, making the heart beat faster. It is so loud that I can hear it in my entire living room. The brain gets enough oxygen that everything else becomes clear. There is no other beautiful sound that can be heard in my body. It's like the perfect meeting of soul and spirit. I cannot explain what is happening inside of me.

My mind only thought about the future. What would be the final day before Aaron leaves? I stood up and began walking the hallway. I couldn't stay still. The pack of cigarettes was on my table. I opened it with one deep breath. "Thank goodness we had only one left!" I told myself. Then I lit up a cigarette and opened the window to let the cool rain droplets wash over my face. The rain today may be wonderful for him, just as it is for me. Call him and say that loudly.

Like her, today I also walked in the rain... When I heard it, wet and scared, I put my head in, shut the window and remained silent. Was it someone I knew?

I'm terrified. At that moment, I didn't expect anyone. They might have been mistaken, I thought. Maybe it is Michael. He is the only one who could have surprised me in such a situation. The knock came again and I was waiting for it. It rang with the door again. I opened it and thought, who is it? The door rang again and I opened it very quickly to see who was there.

It was impossible. It was Sophia ...! The door was AaAaron. I opened it and said hello to him, without inviting him inside. Rain had soaked him, and his eyes were teary. Aaron covered his eyes with his hand, started to straighten his hair and wiped away the tears. He then walked into my living room. The door was the only thing that separated us. I felt him, his breathing, and I'm sure he did too.

Aaron replied, "I thought you wouldn't open the door so I wrote in a note everything I wanted to say."

I said to him, "Please, Aaron, the situation is out of control." "There are certain situations I would like to avoid," I told him. Take this letter. This situation was never under my control. I, unlike you, have never attempted to control it." he replied. In fact, what I really wanted was the opposite. As he talked, I was enraptured by every word. At that time, he stood up and supported the letter with his hand.

Aaron was walking away as I took the letter. I didn't have a clue what to say. I had to close my eyes and take it.

Then I said, "Wait... please tell me where you are going?" I'm going to home ...!" But... but how? "Please tell me what you do." He turned and wiped his tears again, then grabbed my arm, saying;

You slept well tonight ...! A special feeling is sweeping my chest. I haven't been able to sleep for all of this time. "Come on Aaron." I pulled him in by his hands. We were unable to speak, neither him nor me, in the living-room. He stood up and I was in a chair I had forgotten was there. I did not have the nerve to look at him.

It dawned on me that I had to confront the problem. Nothing was easy in front of him. Although I wanted to remain there for as long as I possibly could, I couldn't ignore reality. I didn't believe in miracles. I was told by my heart to be happy and disappointed in the memories that came from my mind. The ice between us was broken when I said, "Aaron you do not look good, you seem tired." As I was running out of breath I went to the window. It was obvious that what I had said made no sense, but I felt the need to speak out or else we'd end up spending the night in silence.

He looked at me in a desperate way after taking a breath. "Can you sit down?"

Without answering his question, I jumped up with a flurry of speed. It seemed to be nothing when I looked at it. Sophia - Yes, sit down. I replied quickly, moving my hands away from the couch. "Sophia I am completely soaked from the rain. A chair would work better for me," he said.

As I recalled Jame's remarks, I replied: "No dear. You can sit on your couch." Aaron was a man in front of me who had the warmth for the home. His mood seemed to be restored by my smile, and his eyes took on a new hue. The man tried to get comfortable, but couldn't. In a quiet voice, he said: "At the very least, you could put a small towel on your couch". The towel cabinet was in the bedroom. I grabbed the largest one and put it on the sofa.

With a smile, I told him: "Now I hope you feel comfortable." He seemed to sink into the sofa, as though he was finally finding comfort. The topic on which we faced each other was brought up. "I didn't want to provoke your anger, but from the email you sent me it appears that I did." In that moment, I was the person who had played with him daily, smiled and controlled everything. But today, he was sitting on my sofa.

No one is able to arouse anger within me. Moreover, you... This situation is out of my control, and it's driving me insane. For the first time ever, I have made friends. I even smiled back at them. Aaron's expression changed. I didn't know what was wrong. He looked sad.

Then, "Am I not too much?" "Should I go?" He asked. As I realized that my words had a lasting impression on him, I replied "Here come with me." In a cheerful smile I offered my hand. He quickly grasped it and squeezed, hoping that he wouldn't let go. I presented him with my tree and opened the window. Do you know that I named him, gave him an extremely special name? Life. "Don't stare at me that way, I am not insane, no!"

No, I don't look at you as if you are crazy. "I realized my thinking was wrong. It just makes me calmer," he replied with sparkling eyes. "I gave her a name I thought was the best. Perhaps not? It has the best name. Every morning when I walk up to the window, he greets me. Oh, I forgot. I once met an elderly man, all thanks to the Life. "How do I get here now? "Is this normal?" He asked.

As I moved away from the glass, I replied "Yes. It is normal given my circumstances." Shaking my hand, he said, "I'm sorry Sophia.

I didn't mean to bother you." "Aaron, Aaron, dear Aaron. "Aaron, Aaron, dear Aaron," I smiled and interrupted. I asked him to come back to the couch, closed the windows and went into the kitchen corner to make a cup. Both of us needed it.

As I made the tea I thought how amazing this was. How can my life be so messed up? This is not possible, I must go back to how I was a couple of days ago. It felt as if I were going crazy. It was like I couldn't feel or connect with anyone. How can I escape this circumstance, where I was being forced to take a path that I did not want? Then I switched to the work conversation. Aaron, we need to discuss it now. "Tell Me, I am ready to answer everything. "I haven't figured out the reasons for your leaving. I think it's a random act. "You aren't like that. Why would you act like that?" I asked.

His face was calmer again when I held the cup. It was obvious what he thought. While I talked to him about my work, he was trying to get me to hug and throw the cup out the window. The cup was in his shaking hand. He placed it on the desk. It's a long time, and you're not going to leave without telling me what your decision is, so I told him while I was drinking tea. Sophia, you're not here for me to discuss work or things you did not understand. Or better yet what you do NOT want to understand. "I came here to tell you how I truly feel about you.

I can no longer have you as a picture in my mind." He drank the tea I made for him and looked at me with tears in his eyes. The whole thing had become history. He began to talk with me. Everything began the day after we first met. The day before I was supposed to make a decision, I called a competing company and it sounded tempting. I didn't know, however, why my first phone call with you made me decide to show up. When I entered the office to do the interview I had no idea what was going on. Even the details are still fresh in my mind. "What was I wearing?" I smiled and asked. "No, nothing. The perfume that you wore on that particular day still lingers in my memory. I felt a strange sensation spread through my entire body. Then I shut my eyes for just a moment and I heard a voice inside telling me to keep this odd smell forever!" "Now, I'm the one who is crazy." He laughed.

"Not at any time, but ..." he interrupted me once again. In a determined voice, he said: "Please hear me to the end." It was clear that he had a better feeling. He sat down on the couch. In his movements and eyes, I could tell that he thought it was the last and first time he would have an opportunity to talk.

I interrupted him several times because I did not want to be involved with his words as much as I wanted to. It was hard for me to admit to myself that I wanted to stop the conversation and hug him forever.

It was a feeling that I couldn't explain, but I could only feel it. I had no power to stop it, or even understand it. When I left the meeting, I took the steps because I didn't want to lose any of the breath that I still had. My hands were totally blocked. I remember starting the car, and the keys falling on the floor at my feet. I tried to reach out with my right hand, while holding my left grip on the steering and foot on brakes, but nothing happened. My emotions were overwhelming and the steering wheel took me with it. The steering wheel took my head with it, my emotions had overwhelmed me.

What's going on with me, come on? That day, I thought to myself: "What's happening?" It's hard to remember exactly how long I was like this, but I do recall that at some point I realized that I looked very clean from where I stood on the 10th floor. I lifted my head and took the keys out of the ignition, started the car, then drove home. The next night, I lay on my sofa in thought and tried to figure out what was going on in my body ...! It's impossible to understand! You are the reason I am in your company and you're always in my sight. When you smile, I am filled with joy. With that, I altered the stream of my thoughts - good morning dear Aaron! These gestures, and some words have been my food up to now.

When was the last time I stopped to tell you what's really going on? I was sometimes even angry, because it appeared to me as if you had done it deliberately! Dear Aaron?! What does this mean dear? How many times have I heard you say "dear?" Yes, it was my intention. It was true, it's what I did. It had an effect that I was aware of.

Aaron's gaze was on me. I could not help but think about myself. Perhaps I did it too much? Perhaps I played on his emotions? The phone interrupted my thoughts, and I had no idea where it was. He was under the couch when I finally found him. It looked like he had sat down there to avoid disturbing us. Sophia: It's Aaron. Doesn't he even know that you are here? As usual, I only thought of hiding the truth. Aaron: No, absolutely not. I completed at the time I set, and I drove you to your home as I do every day, but today I took a different route. He replied firmly. I answered the phone without even knowing why the call was made. Sophia - Hi Henry. Henry: Hi Sophia! How are you doing? Sophia: I feel much better. Thank you for showing interest. I forgot that I was not feeling well, and I hadn't shown up to work. Henry could call me to ask for what? - What did you say to yourself? Henry - You asked me how I felt. I wanted you to feel well. Please say hi to Aaron. I still haven't thanked him for all his hard work.

Sophia: Yes, I agree. When I have the opportunity, I'll thank him. His professionalism has always been based on the truth. Henry:

Then go to bed and tell me how you are doing. Sophia: Yes, Henry. Thanks, too. Aaron was in my face and I was not good. I remembered the entire phone conversation. Why should Aaron be thanked? I had a thousand thoughts - did anyone even know Aaron was with me? I thought I was losing Aaron's trust.

Aaron had a different view. This phone call destroyed all of his plans. It was obvious that he expected me to focus my attention on the business discussions. But in reality, I didn't do that. The words stuck in my mouth when I saw his anxious face. The words wouldn't come out of my mouth. Aaron took up the position in front to make sure he didn't waste any time saying what he had to that evening! Aaron, I understand that you want to discuss work at the moment. But I came to your home to speak to you about it. I did this to prevent another day of feeling that pain that has accompanied me for 8 months. During working hours, I'm sure I wouldn't have the courage to do this! You may not have heard everything I've said, but it is clear that you understand what my situation is. This can't continue ...! Normaly, it's all my fault. Maybe I ate myself, even though the voice in my head told me: Aaron, You will never get what you want.

Sophia, stop asking me. This day is too special for me to go back to the office. Now let me go.

Thank you. He opened the front door with tears in his eyes. It was as though my heart were bursting out. He decided after a year to make his own decisions. It was my fault that I caused him so much hurt, and it wasn't accidental. I knew what he thought of me. It was unbelievable that I used his emotions for my work. As I was following him, I began to feel guilty. It was the shortest corridor in my house ever! I stood up and went towards him. I was trying to stop him...

He hugged me despite the obvious pain in his eyes. In his hands, I felt the warmth of my face. Looking into his eyes, he told me: Aaron-I wish you everything good in your life ...! We all want to experience the life-changing embrace. A warm hug has always meant and expressed more to me than any gesture or words. It would have been nice if it had never ended, but I knew I'd never forget that moment. I wanted to feel so safe in his arms. We would have heard our heartbeats, it was only natural. But neither of us had the strength to hold on forever. As if trying to conceal the tears, I turned around and left.

The door was frozen shut. As he walked away, I only saw his back. My knees buckled as soon as I opened the door. My head was resting on both my knees and the floor. I didn't stop sobbing. It was the same day again. I can't remember where I was when I went to bed. This was not the tomorrow I wanted. But I still had to get to work.

This morning I did not even drink my coffee or go to the window. You were directed to the coffee shop below your workplace. The coffee was so good that I did not want to leave it. I knew I would never find Aaron at the office. I also didn't expect to hear Aaron's voice coming through my glass office. He wouldn't even be in the office when I looked around...but I had to leave.

As soon as I walked into the office I called the director. In a hushed voice I told him about AAaron's departure. There was silence for a few seconds, and I was hoping he could find better words than me. But he couldn't. Sophia: Hello Director, today I went back to work but unfortunately I have bad news. Henry: Sophia, how are you? Sophia - Not even worse, Aaron has resigned. Henry: How can it be? What was it? He did not know how to begin or end. Sophia: I'm not even sure what the reason is (laughing as my tears and spit rolled down my cheeks)! It was a bright morning, the sun shining through my office window. The rain from yesterday was gone, it seemed to be a blizzard for the nature. It was so gloomy that I couldn't feel the sun's rays. Aaron was not visible when I looked up from time-to-time! The heartbeats brought a lot of happiness to me. I couldn't cry because I was working. Aaron was exactly where I am today. I have thought of him for the past eight months. He was without hope, and I had to hold back my emotions.

This feeling can make the heart sad, and even affects the brain. It makes vision and concentration gloomy. It can make the mind and heart gloomy and cause concentration and vision to be dreary. Nothing has any color. Strong people, and those that should be in these situations, are left with only one thought: When will this all end? You would love to be in that exact moment on the day that everything ends! No, this would also not go by without leaving a lasting impression... In the mornings, I would talk to my tree, telling her of the bad luck I had, but also that it had made a lasting impression on me. I said this because I had seen how she was affected by the same thing.

Even though I've been doing interviews for a week now, none have convinced me. They didn't prepare as well. He was always in my mind, writing and returning to his job. I'd be more sensitive to his feelings and I wouldn't treat him that way... I prayed he'd forget, and return as soon as he could. This place belonged to him, and no one could take it. During the week, I was a very bad person. I cried a lot in the car, just like Aaron. I would call Aaron under the pretense of being at work. But I really wanted to listen to his voice and convince him to return, not because I needed him, but to be with me. Sophia, what's the matter with you? I wondered from time-to-time. Was it love or something else? If it's love, then I haven't tried it. It seemed that after five years, I had accepted love.

The feeling of love was something I allowed myself to explore! After deciding to devote myself to only work for the past five years, I worked in the same place and was professional accomplished. But after these five years I felt that I needed to feed my soul, just like trees. The trees cannot live without air and need rain to nourish and sustain them.

It's Friday and I haven't seen my family in a whole month. I called my dad. My father was an idol. He taught me through his actions and not just words, that hard work and honesty are the key to living a peaceful and happy life. He has been working all of his life. The decades are not the same. My father has endured and overcome all the political changes. He is now enjoying retirement, and so am I. He tells me I'm the most important person in his life, but I apologize and I repeat, my mother is more valuable to him. Home has always been my refuge in the darkest times of my life. Where better to forget all your worries, pains, and stress than the bosom of the family... I wanted the opportunity to let Aaron go. He wouldn't come back. It wasn't necessary to live in the hope that he would come back... Both of them were very important to me. Dad: Sophia, your mom is sick, and she's missing you. You should make her happy by giving her a call. Sophia: Dad, although I was very busy for a while, now that things are a bit more stable, I promise to call and visit you often. We have a new contract with our client for three more years.

Sophia: Yes, I spent my entire life educating you in this way and you now complain. Let's not rush, son of a father. The pillar in my house was my father. I can't even imagine the world with him. His solutions and words were always the best for any given situation. He was my idol, and I wanted to be just like him. He was very aware that I only met him when I had been really bad. He knew me and played the part of someone who didn't know. We understood as men very well in silence, and we also knew that they were white lies. My mother was not available to me. Since the loss of my sister she has been ill. I feel the same way. But I've convinced myself that her presence is with me. My mother was devastated when she lost my sister. I tried to help her cope for years, but it only made things worse. She loved me so deeply that she could hear my voice on the telephone.

When I look at the photo in my childhood bedroom, my sister Ellen is still there, and I'm very young... It hurts me to see it but I didn't want it ruined, so I let it stay. In their home, when I go to sleep, I don't turn the lights off. I am left feeling very lonely and my memories of Ellen are brought back. For him, these photos are very important. I'd rather suffer for my mother than myself. It's different today, when I looked at the pictures, my feelings changed. I felt even worse. I thought I had begun my fortune at an early age like my "life tree".

I found it terrible that you have lived with your sister for 15 years and then find out about it only in a photo. Today I really missed Ellen, and I began to feel my mother's sorrow more. It was much bigger than the feelings I felt when I first entered the room. Sophia - Father, please leave the suitcase and hug your dad. You haven't been with him for a month. Does it seem right to spend time in this room?

He denied the pain and appeared stronger...but that was not true. It is often the strongest who appear to be most vulnerable. I too looked like him. I had a mountain inside of unlived emotions and words that were unbreakable. Then, I thought of Aaron. Maybe he was part of those feelings. Or maybe I'm wrong ...? Sophia: I came to greet my king, and hugged him. He moaned. Father: My Princess, I'm not old enough to bear this hug. You will one day die for me. My mom was my closest friend and I could not sleep that night alone. I asked her to be near me.

Ellen stayed with us all night, we talked, laughed, and it was as though Ellen were with us. I told my mother about all of the wonderful moments I had with Ellen, including how I burst into laughter a great deal. Everything is always perfect in my mother's home, the orderliness and cleanliness, not to mention, of course, the delicious food. My mother woke me up early and had already prepared my breakfast. She had also taught me to always eat the breakfast.

It was important. Even though I woke up early, my mother had gotten up before me, she prepared breakfast for me, and taught that it was important to eat this meal.

You saw it wasn't the proper form to bring up Ellen again. The tobacco store was not close and I needed to go by car because I missed cigarettes. My father was amused when I said I would be buying poison. I have always made this joke. I felt better. Aaron was gone, but the warmth of my family may have helped me to forget him and feel better. On the radio, the lyrics of the songs put me in deep thoughts! Then I stopped the car, greeted the residents in the café with my head and looked to the left to see if I could cross the street.

I was able to do so because the traffic had stopped. My eyes were rubbing and I called out to my brain because I could not believe what I saw. Aaron, are you in front of my face? Aaron is his name. "You said it to yourself!" Aaron is opening his eyes, trying to determine if I am dreaming or not. What is he trying to say? Was he following me? The man was sitting in front of a morning cup of coffee with a paper and looked as though he'd been awake for many nights. With a surprised look, he put the paper down and said: AAaron- Sophia? !

It was probably the opportunity that both of us were waiting for. You followed me, both of us said with an open smile and voice that showed our distress. Aaron: No Sophia. I moved to this side. I had an interview for a job today. I was a few kilometers away from my destination, but I felt tired so I decided to sit down and have a cup of coffee. Sophia: You're going to have an interview on Saturday? Sophia - You have an interview this Saturday? Aaron - I do have Hene but I've booked a hotel a few kilometres away. I wanted to get a feel for the area, and see if it was something I liked. I am looking for a home... Shortly, I am looking to move away from my current location.

I had a good knowledge of the region, and I wanted to find out where he would be doing the interview. I was interested in anything... He could not do it. Aaron - What about you? Aaron - Sophia, I was born right here. My parents are often here, but my home is higher, and not the middle.

I also live in an area where air quality is better for me, as my lungs have been damaged by city pollution. I turned to go. It was not possible for him to act in that way! I had accepted it as a part of me! Aaron: Please, don't go, come sit with me, we'll talk. Drink something... Sophia I miss you. Sophia: No, thank you. I've got more important things today.

Aaron: I'm sorry, but you were blind. I did make a mistake with you in the office one year ago and was no longer interested. Sophia's love is not like any other, and it can't even be described. I must leave. When I heard these words, I felt both happy and sad. He was speaking about the past. It seemed that he forgot me, before you. I appeared to be a distant memory. Sophia: I'm wishing you the best for Hena even though I haven't found out the distance from your current workplace. I was determined to find out where Hena would be going for her interview.

Aaron - I congratulate you. Sophia, what are you saying? Sophia, I believe in you. The information was given to me and I was aware of his location at Henen. However, I did not know the time that he was scheduled for the interview. I went home quickly, Aaron had disappeared, the chair had been moved so far, it was as though it was gone with the wind. In a town as small as his, my father had worked with nearly everyone in the past. How could I tell my father about the situation? He might not understand if I said the truth. I'd tell him he caused economic harm to us by leaving his job.

Ask my father to help me. If it were possible, I would have my father call that bank right now! Aaron's place was right in front of me, just a glass away, and I didn't want to be miles from him. Aaron's office was nowhere to be found. I knew that I had done something wrong. My father was waiting for me when I got home. I told him I had to speak to him. I then sat in the balcony, my breath keeping me from speaking. My father asked me why my friend had to call him early Monday morning. Aaron shouldn't be allowed to stay there... He smiled and said: Father, my dear daughter! You are an adult now and must know that the intrigues of life won't get you anywhere.

The guy had good reasons for leaving the company, and I believe that they were very compelling. Today, it's easy to get a new job. I doubt that he left without having an interview. Sophia: Dad, are you telling me that he has the job at Henen now? He must have left to get this job, it seems! Sophia - He doesn't, Father, because it is just an interview. So, you need to sit down and think about it.

He knew everything. He understood everything. It was he who taught me the values I hold dear. I did ask him to give up his life on a whim. That night, I kept my eyes open. Tears were often my companion. Aaroni seemed further and farther away. The hope for change was fading. The thought of returning to my home, with the furnishings that I worked so hard to acquire, now seemed worthless, was difficult.

The silence in the house was deafening and I felt sad about returning to an office that had been filled with papers but now seemed empty. Father: "My daughter, do not let your mind overcome your heart. He who acts from the heart always wins." He understood me better than I understood myself. His words told me to not be harsh on myself.

In the past three months I was very busy and there wasn't anyone in front of my desk. Aaron's desk was already gone! Ich habe mich consciously overburdened. Aaron's work was something I wanted to take on myself. Aaron is someone I do not know. He may work in my hometown. I've been to my parents three times already this month, and my luck hasn't been great. What happened during the interview is not of interest to me. The memories of him were fading, maybe I didn't have time, because the bank was closed on the weekends. My mind often told me to go and check if Aaron started working at the bank. It was like the memories were fading away, perhaps I did not have the time. I was so busy with my work that I drowned myself in it.

It was so gorgeous, even with the darkness surrounding it. The stars were shining brightly. When I saw her, I was filled with deep thoughts. It seemed like she'd found love, and she appeared to be happy. A gentle breeze caressed her lcaves. That is when I asked her.

You who are older, who has been through and faced more than I have... show me what you have done. What is love, tell me the truth? I heard a voice inside tell me that love is pain. You cannot see it, touch it and find it. It does happen! This happens to fathers, mothers, Ellen... T

he word "love" for Aaron would not leave my mind, nor could I say it out loud. It was as though Life were looking me in the eye, and it appeared to be saying that you are spoilt by beauty, like it had read my mind, but didn't agree! Closed my eyes, Life replied: "Be like me. I experience every emotion in my lifetime. I am not tired in rain, snow or heat.

The woman did it, went through all the difficulties with courage and this made her stronger. She picked flowers again in spring... what am I doing? I want to get away! Mental burdens over the past few months caused me to lose some weight. I didn't know whether it was Aaroni or work, but I knew my father would be very unhappy if he saw me like this. Mom would be even more upset, as she could not tolerate the slightest hint of flu from me...

How could I? It was important to me that I find someone else in the office. Take some time off, and recover my weight. Even though I thought I would need some therapy sessions, I didn't think I really needed them.

Maybe a psychologist with these skills could help me out of the darkness I was in. But it was all just thoughts. My health was my main concern, so I stopped smoking. I believed that I could recover the weight I lost if I continued to eat regularly, and quit smoking even when I had a busy job. It was obvious that I was slowly killing myself. I was not helped by my past. After Ellen's passing, I felt a great deal of loneliness. My thoughts often return to me. The pain in my parent's eyes made me hide my emotions.

My eyes were closed and I spitted and cried through my teeth, never letting the tears or spittle escape. My tears came out at night and I breathed with my mouth to make sure that no one could hear that my nose had been blocked. It's how I learnt to suffer without anyone feeling it. As I grew older, it became embarrassing to see me crying in front of others. Today was the first time I've ever cried in public. Aaron, today in the office reminded me that days became weeks, and then months, but I did not want those weeks to become years.

He had made a mark on me. I may have loved him just as much as Aaron loved me during the entire time they worked together. Men are more free than women. They have the courage and confidence to express their feelings and to enjoy them. We have to battle with ourselves.

What if AAaron had been my life too? It was obvious that I loved him and liked what I felt... But why didn't I dare to share this with him ...?? The mistake would have been to take a wrong decision and live, rather than be where I am now! It's possible that everything ended the same way as today. He in another country and I here. But, I would not have felt his absence... Or maybe we would still be together.

Sophia, concentrate on your work. Aaron is gone. How many times must I repeat this to myself? Mozart's Symphonies were in my office, so I listened to them. They gave me peace and would help me be more focussed at work. Ellen was always playing Mozart in my head, and I could feel her nostalgia. It could have been that I wanted to avoid work or I wanted to forget Aaron. With Ella's music, though, the thoughts I had didn't disappear, they just became more sweet.

I thought the same thing would happen to the memories of Aaron but, it didn't, Mozart made them bitter. Ellen was a part of my world for over 15 years, and she has only left behind beautiful memories and the pain that her absence has caused ...! Aaron, on the other hand, was a different story. I could not recall anything beautiful about him, nor did I have any fond memories of his. I only had moments that brought me to tears. It was too late to take any medicine, and I did not have the strength to switch off Mozart.

The tears started to flow as I put my hands on the keyboard, hurled the pen, and turned away from the window. But Life wasn't there! Who knows how often Aaron felt empty and alone during his year with us. You said, "I have to find him."

This can't continue. Aaron was not there. He had left after a short time, and he claimed that the work was just too demanding. This time I've lost him. I'd been calm for months, convinced he was working in my hometown bank. Now you have lost him for good - said yourself. After wiping away the tears and removing the disk, I returned to my work with tears. Even the case had no chance... He will be gone. In fact, it is so far gone that the case itself has lost all hope. The elevator man was there to say good morning, and goodbye. I realized he always knew when I entered and left the building. I was able to tell my father about the situation and he asked how frequently we spoke on the telephone. Dad, what do you want to say? I'm waiting. He asked me always smiling.

Sophia: No, Dad, I do not have any news. I will be first to announce when there is a new development. Come on, it's time to leave. This is how I ended the call to prevent my father from saying anything else to me. Aaron has been gone for a year! Aaron was no longer with us. I knew it and had accepted the fact that it would be a distant memory.

But unlike Ellen, Aaron is a lifeless one. So I kept them both in my mind, and I often thought of them. Ellen had left the office at an early age, but all of us continued to live our lives. I brought in another employee in the office, just as I did for Aaron. I put him into a deep drawer in my heart and continued living my life. Daniel should not have sat in the spot where Aaron used to sit, because no one can replace him. So I made another desk opposite.

So, I could control them more effectively, and no one would be able to see me. It was unnecessary for anyone to be in my office. This was the same mistake that I made when Aaron was there. Maybe if I hadn't looked through this mosque each day, nothing would have occurred. Before I met Aaron, I was strong and had gone back to Sophia. Everyone respected me as Sophia and not just as my superior at work. Jeten and I talk every morning. I can see his transformation day-by-day. But I've yet to find the time to meet him. It will be very soon. The mother, after years of therapy, seemed to have found her inner peace. She was happier.

Maybe, like me she kept Ellen's memory alive in her mind, as beautiful and smiling as she once was. I'm not sure how much words my father has, but he is like me when it comes to his spiritual state. He is in good health and I am sure he's strong. Every time I speak to him, I feel unimaginable power.

He seemed to be very concerned about me. A strong cough had been bothering me for about a month. It didn't happen often but yesterday I was talking to my father and he mentioned it. He was worried, so I told him I'd done the check-ups and had no worries.

What is the coughing, Father? Why don't visit? Why don't stop? Never have I heard such an unusual cough. Sophia: You have nothing, dad? What do you mean by that? The doctor had me checked and I followed all his instructions, but there was nothing. This is a cold which will soon pass. You have no idea what we went through in the office when the director, who had lived with his fiancée for seven years, decided to marry her. Daniel, who worked with us for some time, was also invited. All were focused on her look. His marriage seemed to have started just two weeks earlier.

As I listened to the conversation in the office, I wondered how much preoccupation the future wife has for her look. I laughed out loud. The moment I received the invitation, I immediately knew what I would wear. I already had a dress that I hadn't worn in ages, so it was the perfect occasion to debut it. Who knows how long that pink dress will remain in that wardrobe? Not even formal occasions have been my cup of tea. I've only attended them on rare, very important occasions. It's also why I only have a few formal gowns in my closet.

When I was getting ready I took a pair casual shoes along with me. It made me laugh to see myself wearing a dress so beautiful and casual shoes. It was in my mind to do that to make the director laugh and to be able to share a joke with him. But it wasn't the right time. This was his most important day. I needed to show respect to him regardless of our mutual confidence.

Then I closed the vehicle, shut the door, put the high-heeled black sandals on, draped the jacket around my shoulders and led you all to the event. It was the first time I had ever been late. At home, my hair looked awful. I tried several different styles, but in the end I combed it and parted it down the middle. As I climbed the stairs, a light breeze blew through my hair. I found it difficult to see the staircase as I held the can in one hand and removed the hair with my other.

After being about 30 minutes behind schedule, I went straight to my wife's house. Sophia: "Please forgive me. I am sorry. I apologize for the delay." I then took the prepared gift from my bag. I put money into an envelope because I didn't want to miss out on such a moment and choose something special. It was a gift that nobody wanted, but I thought it the least I could give to both of them. They have always been good friends. I've never felt the weight of their friendship, nor have I ever seen them.

I was treated so well by them that my gift seemed insignificant. Sophia: I apologize for my delay, and for how I gave you your gift. I am not a practical person. Sophia would not be my name if I acted like that. We all laughed together. It was obvious that I was doing it wrong, but there was no way to know the correct way. I decided to go ahead and make a mistake rather than wait to ask about how to give gifts to newlyweds.

Everybody was dancing. The director approached me for a moment and said with a smile: Henry - You never go unnoticed. I was approached by the director for a few moments and he said, with a grin: Henry -- You are never unnoticed. Sophia is constantly being asked about what you are doing. -I smiled hesitantly and couldn't find the words to respond. He turned to go but returned with a more serious expression. Henry: Sophia, it looks like not everyone has arrived. He turned away from the door without finishing his sentence and replied: Henry. He left with a smile.

What I saw was a boy tall with black hair. He was beautiful, even more so than last year. As he approached them slowly, he smiled and welcomed them with warmth. The glass of champagne dropped from my hand, I had trembling legs, and no one was in the room for me. Aaron looked better, and he was even smiling.

Aaron talked for quite a while with the director. He destroyed everything that I'd built in this past year. I archived everything into my memory and it all ended then. Once again, strong feelings overtake me. He would go again, I knew. It was just that I thought it would be a while before I could forget him. Aaroni was standing in front me once again. I'd worked hard with my emotions, I fought myself for stability.

Aaron did not even look up while talking with the director. It was a pleasure to look at him head-to-toe. I wanted to hug him and tell everyone about this tough year I had without him. I also wanted to say out loud that I am happy to be seeing him again. However, I chose to go to the bathroom. I didn't stop crying, and I did it as loud as I could. Aaron seemed to forget me. He was superior. He seemed very happy, calm and smiling.

After a few moments, I washed my face with cold water to get rid of any tears. I also had to cover any marks that were on my skin. Then I went up to the director and tried to think of an excuse to leave. You told me I wasn't well. You may have heard me say that my father had called to tell me of an urgent issue... what did I actually tell you? My legs buckled as soon as I took a quick step. I tried to stand up fast, but I only had the meeting with director in mind. I just wanted to leave as quickly as possible.

A hand squeezed on my arm, and it helped me to regain my balance. It was too dangerous to look up to see. I was focused on one thing - to get out as quickly as possible. Aaron: Sophia! You look so beautiful today. It was AAaron's voice! He would have known that I was in tears if I raised my head. Aaron, I'm sorry I didn't say goodbye sooner. I've been looking for you and wanted to greet you. I'm rushing out of time, but couldn't let him go without saying hi. As I tried to cover my eyes by pulling my hair back, he pulled me closer to him. He held me up by my arms and then my hands with one hand.

At that time, he didn't want to look at anything but hug me. We all felt the pain of being apart in our bodies as we clenched up our hands. He hugged me until I forgot about the year that had passed without him. The hug felt like the entire sky was inside me. He did not see the tears on my eyes, and I didn't even see his face. It was impossible for me to remove my head from the shoulder. My hands were around his neck to let him know that I would not be satisfied until I had a good hug. My chest moved, filled up and then deflated. As always, he felt me cry silently in his arms. He squeezed my hard, and also caressed the hair on my neck all the way to my middle back. He squeezed me hard and caressed my hair from the middle of my back to the neck. I heard him urging me on Aaroni - Shshsh ... I'm here. The first time I could not control myself. I didn't think about it, and just wanted to relax in his arms. Even as I sat there, he said in a sweet voice AAaron – Sophia, How are you? It was a simple question, but it took on a real meaning - How did I feel? His question was a real one. Was he asking me how I felt? How was I feeling? What had happened to ...?? Even after I had gotten out of his arm, I could not look him directly in the eyes, so I replied in a quiet voice that I was okay. After I answered, I could hear him laugh.

Aaron - You can't be that good! - In a friendly voice, he told me that I was not feeling well. By bringing my face close to his, I use his right hand. The only way to escape was for their eyes to collide... I continued the sentence. Aaron - Because I talk with the director often, I know about your situation professionally. He tells me you've done very well in this past year. It must have taken you a while to think of doing such a crazy thing. Now I do hope Daniel made it a bit easier for you.

During this hug, I was able to understand your current spiritual condition. - He let me know he was aware of my existence. Aaron was the reason I fell in love. She could transform the way people see things with two words and a hug. With a hug she can change lives, help others, be a guide, etc. It was the one that I needed. Did he understand what I went through this past year?

He was calm and didn't seem to want to bring up topics that could make me feel worse. It seemed like he already knew what I felt, but he wanted to show concern for me. He talked to me as though he were a professional. He spoke about many professional subjects, but I did not tell him his workplace! The bank in my hometown came to mind. Sophia: I learned that you don't work with us at the bank. Aaron - Aaron, how do you know? Sophia: Everyone in the small town knows everyone else, so they all know my father, and I too.

Aaron - So, in a few sentences, they answered your question about me? Sophia: No, no I didn't hear it at the cafés in the city. Aaron: How odd, I only stayed for one week before I left... I found the city too sad for me. He placed his mouth on the accelerator. My mind said it would be better to not know. I didn't have the courage to inquire about his current job. He had clearly forgotten about me. It was evident on his face. Aaron said he had a limited time to spare and was leaving, but is still present.

We were all sitting in the front, enjoying this momentous occasion for newlyweds. Aaron was in front of us. Aaron was in front of me, but I could not see. He would soon leave and I might never see him again. I didn't want to share the moment with Aaron. I felt my body shake as our eyes crossed several times. For a moment, it was like it was mine.

In that moment, I couldn't resist. The party went on. I tried to see Aaron but he hadn't returned. The director was relieved when I told him that I would have to leave. I then turned around and walked out. I knew no one else was watching me so it was easy to cry. It will be your longest night ever - I told myself as I walked out. Once I was outside, I could cry freely because no one would see me. My left hand covered my mouth because I did not want to cry. The car appeared to be further away now than it ever was. When I began to descend, I could not see the steps.

The same hand squeezed my arm as I went down the steps. Aaron was waiting outside for me as if knowing I would leave earlier without him. The road diverted and the direction of the vehicle was different. Aaron took deep breaths, didn't say a word to me and never turned his head. I heard his footsteps and could barely keep my heels in place. It was my intention to prevent him from leaving and follow him barefoot but there wasn't time.

I only had to hold his hand. It was around 17:00h when the party started, but it had now become dark and stars began to appear in the night sky. As if praying that the night wouldn't end, I lifted my head. He stopped finally, I couldn't tell where I was and I didn't want to. Before his eyes, nothing existed. Only me, him and a sky filled with stars.

Now that I was able to stand in front of the man, my tears had not dried up and now even more quickly. The car stopped abruptly and without any right. The eyes were not the same as when you first arrived at the party. They looked tired, teary and lacked any sparkle. His tears were quickly dried up. Aaron: What a hard dog! Wiping tears away. The only thing I can't forget is the pain I felt when I listened to Mozart symphonies. I searched the world for healing melodies and sought the advice of experts, but it never worked. Life is the only way to heal. I'm going to try and live that with you. Let's even do it hidden, if it makes you feel better. Give me a chance to do it, and I am sure that it will be so successful you won't believe it. His words were hurriedly spoken, as though he thought it was his last chance to get it right.

When I saw stars smiling and the breeze caressing the hair of my head, I was relieved. Aaron squeezed my hands, as if to ask for approval. He was hoping that a positive word would bring him some hope. I couldn't stand up. I felt paralyzed. Aaron went through the same stages as I did and had never forgotten me. I saw Aaron more in love after this separation of a year. Sophia: Why did you break up with Aaron? We might be very different now! We might have been able to face it together. Aaron, I've suffered greatly with your departure. You are still in my thoughts and heart. Even though the memory is bitter, it will always be there.

Why did Aaron leave you? Why did you hurt me like this? He didn't want to even answer my questions. He was trying to dispel any doubts I had with the facts. So close to him that I could feel his lips on my cheek, I squeezed my face in between his palms. My feelings and everything else was surrendered to him.

He also thought that this moment was a fantasy, so he grabbed me by the throat to show that it wasn't a nightmare. My right hand swept across my face, stopping at my lips. His gaze seemed to be a part of my pulse. The reality around me was gone and I lived only this dream, which I never wanted to end. My thumb touched my lips, and our eyes fused together... We had only one goal in that moment. Aaron: I've waited so long for today, Sophia. The words became a kiss.

My heart was bursting out of my chest. I kept opening my eyes, letting him taste the kiss. As he pulled my head onto his shoulder I felt safe, even though I shook all over. He held his head and brought me close to his body with one hand. Even though I was on his shoulder, I could still hear his heartbeat. The words came to me as he squeezed and hugged me. Aaron, My Angel Sophia. Music could be heard all the way up where we stood. Aaron sang to me with a soft voice, as though he was singing me lullabies. Now I was in Aaron's arms, it was magical.

It was as if my thoughts had disappeared and I could fly with him. On his special day, even the director couldn't be more happy than us. I felt as though the party was planned for us both. My soul danced! My life has been filled with too many hardships and I've had to make some drastic choices for me. My parents, who both worked hard, held high-ranking positions at work.

We have always been at the center, and we've been envied by others. After Ellen died, I found it very hard. After her death, everything seemed like a joke to each other. I can tell you that people were not even sorry for Ellen's passing! After her funeral, she cried the first time. Maybe it was because of Ellen's passing, but this is the first I have seen of her. People started talking and talking out of context about her: what did he to that a 15-year old child would die? We don't have enough food to feed him and he has plenty of money for the burial!

It was not subtle. It was to demonstrate his state. Sophia was taught how to cry. She looked heartless and cried as an actor would. ? ! How many sentences caused my father's tears to fall and he didn't even try to hide from us... They did not know that the eyes cry when the heart cries... Or maybe they were aware but did it deliberately. They have changed my life in such a way that it is now apparent to you. They were both always prepared:

My mother would often leave her job to join her friends on a night out. I recall that she once took some money out of a pocket in one of her skirts. It is dry, and I give it to a neighbor. He would probably have requested it. I was still young, but I knew that the family's economic condition was poor. Father hosted many people in his home.

The people who lived near the road and didn't have money for even the most basic hostel were those that had to stay there. She was intolerant, cooking for them even at midnight, feeling sorry for her, but not even thinking about taking time off for herself. Even though she had to get up early the next morning for work, I saw the sparkle in her eye when she prepared the food, as if she wanted at least a little break from their urine .....

My school life was also very difficult. I had to deal with a lot of criticism from my peers, who couldn't accept the way I expressed myself. But I never gave up, because I wasn't alone, didn't have any friends, and hadn't made enemies. It was then that I lost all faith in humanity, yet never any kindness. I have always helped those in need, just as my parents did. My smile has never been taken from me. The good word, education, culture and culture for all. Life was no longer there to keep me company. Triny was my cat until I graduated. She left just as I began my studies at university.

It's been ten years since she became my friend. At first, there was two of us. She seemed to have suffered less than I did when Ellen died, or perhaps she helped me because she is strong. I had no friends in high school. I only started making friends during university. It was a mixture of envy, from the study of who had done it better to who received more marks, or who was the teacher's favorite. Such things were enjoyable for me. I was surrounded by many acquaintances, but I only had one close friend. I was always able to get along with men.

I was confident that I was someone they would want to spend the rest of their lives with. It was a two-year love affair, if you can call it such. Maybe because I only tried love a year before, I've never felt disappointed. I have made decisions based on my feelings being frozen from other disappointments. Never have I allowed myself to be tempted. Nothing would ever lead me anywhere. The ending of many of my cases was less than satisfactory. Shortly, I have learned from other people's mistakes...

Gabriel and I are very close friends today because I treated everyone with kindness and was good to him before and after we started dating. Respect is better than love, or even physical attraction. The passion that we shared at the time.

It just so happened that I was with him and his family when he started a family. I love seeing him happy even though I knew that he wanted someone like me to be close by him.

Gabriel was not less important than Anna, but I felt that Anna deserved more.

Truthfully, I've been through a lot. I was in bigger situations than I could handle and yet I still managed to succeed. Today, I am sorry about all I've been through. I had the right too to experience all stages of my life the way nature intended. No, that wasn't feasible - I was a teenager and had to face problems no one else has ever faced. Well, I tell myself that today you will be forgiven all your wounds. Perhaps I look better to the world, with my scars, than Life does.

Aaron brought back all of my memories the minute he took me into his arms. It was as though I had downloaded and left all my emotions from the past in his arms. They no longer belonged to me. Aaron made me forget my past in that moment.

Aaron: "Sophia, I'm in love with you. I love Sophia." While holding his head.

Sophia - Thank you, Aaron!

Aaron, I also love you - now I realize that maybe I have loved him from the very first day...

Aaron: Don't say that you can't contact me tomorrow. I will go where I am from, and you are going to continue staying locked up at the office or home.

Sophia: No Aaron! Maybe tonight, a new light of hope will shine for both you and I. Aaron thought my answer was unbelievable, that I would allow him to call me the next day, and to have us both live together, experiencing this emotion... Sophia: After all, love ...- is essential to life. Aaron: I would like to go with you. Sophia: Yes, my car is here, but how do we get there? Aaron: Let me lead you to the brightest star in this evening by driving ahead of you. - He said kissing me again. We were caught in traffic and we were heading to our cars.

Aaron was in the lead, while I followed behind. You did a good job, even though I may have made a mistake on my way home. While driving, my mind was only on his kiss. Aaron was an absolute gentleman. I felt bad that we were so far apart and had spent over a year without each other. Aaron emerged from the car, walked up to me and kissed me deeply. Aaron: Sophia, it's not something I want to do but I must, I just know that I will. Sophia- Natan- Aaron- Sophia, I answered you in a way that I'm not sure if you heard.

My legs fell off, I fell to the corridor floor, and I was drowned by my thoughts. I shut the door. I then knew no one had seen me. It wasn't all a nightmare, Aaron had returned, the carpet was extra-soft, the furniture was shining, and I could see that the whole living room was shining. My hands were touching my lips as I kissed the entire house to recall the taste of Aaron's kiss. Then I went to sleep.

When I woke up, it was 3:00 AM. Sophia, get up Sophia! You said to yourself as you directed you towards the bed. The pink dress was on my bed that night and I did not feel anything. This was the first day in six years I had not shown up to work. No one knew about it. It was my third fall in as many days. I never fell before, and I always had control over myself. From where I stood, I knew that today was a lost cause.

The time was 10:10 in the morning. I picked up the phone, and it rang 3 times without me hearing it. What do I do? "What should I do?" I asked myself. Daniel was the person who answered when I dialed the office. Daniel: Sophia, no worries, we are all more or less in the same position. We're walking about the office holding coffee, and we seem to be more focused. He laughed. Sophia: No Daniel. I said that I would be prepared in an hour and present myself at the office. You have covered my work for many hours.

Then I stood up, walked to the mirror and began to remove my dress. It would be the most beautiful thing I have ever worn. 'Today is different, I told myself. After removing my dress, I put it in a shelf and took a shower with half-wet hair. The bed had never been unmade before. I quickly dressed and left. My face looked comical but I noticed that my eyes shone. I also liked Sophia, who was half-wet and had her hair in a bun. No time today for my black eye pencil, or lipstick. Even better, the smell and color of Aaron's kiss could not be replaced by any lipstick. The beautiful music on the radio and the reflection in the mirror made my eyes sparkle.

Sophia: Daniel, please forgive me, I have no idea why I am not awake. You heard me, and my alarm went off. My phone rang 3 times. I directed you back to the office and laughed. It was a good day at work. I could not wait to get out. I did not take any time off that day to make up for the lateness. I also wanted to finish the day quickly and do things I had planned to do tomorrow. The working day was now free, and I took the time to reflect on Aaron's death, what happened yesterday, Mozart's Symphonies seemed more beautiful than ever... my father taught me to listen to classical music all of his life. He always said: "He is a healer, friend, in any circumstance." (he was correct). After I had finished my work, I went to leave the office. I caught a cold and stopped in the elevator to rest.

The elevator was full when I got in, and to my surprise the exact same man entered at the same moment as me. Zorteria: Hello Sophia! Today you look more beautiful than ever. Sophia smiled and said, "Thank you Lord!" I turned my back and answered. He complimented my face today, when I wasn't feeling well. My face was apparently more beautiful today than it had ever been. I knew the real beauty comes from within. My face was pale as I walked to the parking area to retrieve the car, and then home.

All day, Aaron was on my mind, but now he wasn't. He could call me... perhaps he was trying to be respectful of my schedule or maybe like me, he had a late start? He might still be at work... Silently, I answered my logical instinct which often disturbs me! I was at home and everything looked more attractive to me. Even the decor of my house felt comfortable. With a smile I looked out of the window, and I pointed you towards Life.

Sophia: I'm sorry, but I have no idea what to say. It's hard to know what to say... I seem to be in blooming season too, like you, and I am just as happy... I went silently over everything that happened to me the previous night, making comparisons to him often to try to understand what had occurred!

Aaron had not been heard. He was very familiar with me and knew I never had called him. I knew he would lead me down the road of emotions. His gesture was completely inappropriate because I could not give any commands. As I usually do, I didn't think in a negative way. The ringing phone interrupted my thoughts. It was the director. I received this unexpected call, he left on his honeymoon. What could have happened to him?

Sophia, Director: Hello, What happened? Is there anything wrong?

Henry - Sophia, calm down! Take a deep breath. Nothing happened. You will be opening the office tomorrow at 9 am. There is some work being done, and I was told that it will take an extra hour to finish everything.

Sophia: I'm with you, but... I couldn't make out anything when I wrapped the paper around my nose.

Henry: But tomorrow, at 9 am, and not 8 pm, you'll sleep more. He laughed.

Sophia: Okay then, have a great honeymoon. I wish you both the best.

The man was working in his office, and I did not know what he was doing.

Danieli was not aware of the changes that took place during my two-hour delay.

It was strange, I thought.

Aaron was still not listening to me. I had a phone call that took a couple of minutes away, but then brought him back. Aaron didn't seem to be listening and I did not want to spend another night in mental exhaustion, living with the fear that Aaron might leave again.

I decided, yes yes, to go to the party if it was possible. Wasn't it the opportunity that brought us together last night? And where was Aaroni at the wedding of the director when I thought about that? It's possible that another opportunity will arise tonight. Maybe Aaron will be heading my way and I see him in the street. I might end up meeting them in the city outside in a café.

At that time, my thoughts were interrupted. Aaron was most likely far from the city and he may have left again this time. I carried on walking until I got to the café with the transparent windows. They were so transparent, you could not tell whether they were present or absent.

Only the city lights and stars shone. I chose to sit inside because I'm used to seeing through glass. There was nobody inside and everyone was outside.

It was enough to watch them talk and smile, not to listen to their words.

In my lifetime, I've managed to listen to people and understand their words without really listening. Their gestures, facial expressions and movements are all I need to know. This helped me to see what was in front of me, as well as how to behave.

Aaron was standing before the window for over a year, and I never understood his personality. Aaron was the only person I knew whose personality I could only understand when he talked. He was also one of few that I didn't just understand by his everyday gestures and behavior. In my mind, I finished drinking the juice that I ordered. I then headed home. My legs seemed to be walking themselves. I looked down at them, and laughed, because I'd never felt lighter. Some people returned home on foot while others took public transportation, or by vehicle.

The phone was still dead. Then I turned on the lamp and read until I fell to sleep. As usual, the bell rang, so I had a bit more time to prepare. In fact, I spent all of my time in front the mirror. Although I did not change my appearance, I still liked seeing myself and the sparkle in my eye. Aaron wasn't even living, but his memories, taste of lips and the events that happened had made me feel sweet.

It's possible that he won't be around for long, but I have enough wonderful memories of him to last more than one day. What will tomorrow bring without you? I did not want to close myself off to the feeling which had been with me for over a year.

Even today, I don't know how I managed to sing all of those songs I heard that day in the car. Sometimes, even the lyrics I did not understand. As always, the same guy in the elevator. But this time, I was one hour late. What made his existence possible today? "I asked myself, surprised! Sophia: Hello Arnold! Do you have any work today at the office? I asked him. After a brief pause, he could not find the right words to say, but eventually he found them and replied. Arnold:

No, Sophia. I have no idea what you're talking about. I am late for work today. Sleep, sleep. - Smiling. He knows I didn't believe him. After a friendly greeting, I left the elevator. He confirmed that the office's location was such that I could easily access it from the outside of the building. Now I am unsure about the hours he works. -I laughed, and pointed you towards the automatic office door. It was interesting to see and hear about the work that had been done in my absence. My office wasn't far away from the entrance, but I couldn't find it until after turning to the left and doing a 180-degree turn.

At first you couldn't tell that anything had changed. Where did these works take place? What changes have been made? This game is not very fun? You were directed to my office by me as I talked to myself. With all my curiosity, I walked and thought. It was the same as my office, and it did not change. It was a shock to me when I saw that a decision had been taken without consulting with me. He had to not only get my approval or inform me but also implement it now, for over a year. You thought to yourself. It was real, so I sped up to confirm what I saw with my own eyes. Someone had the guts to rebuild a fully functional desk in front of my office! The computer was running and all the papers on the desk were warm.

Then I told you to come into the office. I took a deep breath and threw my can onto the chair of my desk. And then, with my phone, grabbed it.

The director could have told me this once, but I kept repeating it myself.

Aaron was the only person who could be seen. The manager was not available when I called. I immediately dialed his number without hesitation. I then hung up and began to remove my jacket. I felt very angry. Maybe the manager no longer considered me and that the decisions were made by myself.

He should have told me. With all my anger, I took off my bag, hung up the jacket and sat on the chair. It would have been best if I hadn't picked up the bag. I was just lowering my head to switch on the computer. Aaron is standing in front of my desk with a tray and a suit on, as he always does during work hours.

Aaron's back was pushing my transparent office door as I sat with my hands on the power button on my computer. I could not even speak.

Aaron: Last time, we began with tea. Today I believe it is time to begin with coffee. As if to bring my reality back to me, he kissed my cheeks with sweetness, delicacy and strength.

Aaron: Good morning, dear. Do you like our surprises? He said to me, and then sat in front of my face.

Why was Aaron speaking in the crowd then? What else was there to know? It was important to me that no one knew I had fallen in love.

Sophia: What Aaron is talking about? What about the other people who share our emotions? I felt guilty for all the people who knew how much Aaron meant to me.

Aaron: When will your mind begin to follow the heart? Will you stay the same forever? You should be known to the whole world! He smiled and let me know that my attitude needed to be changed now.

The whooping-cough, as I call it, won't allow me to respond with my usual irony. With a strong cough, I got to the bathroom. I was embarrassed in front of him.

Closed the door, I felt at ease to allow the cough to take me as it pleases!

The pain was unusual. I reflected on everything in that brief time before the mirror, and even tried to make my face look better.

Aaron approached me quickly as soon I emerged from the door.

Aaron: This isn't normal. Please promise that you will come and see me to find out why.

Sophia: Aaron, I'm done with these jokes. Please continue your work.

Aaron: Don't ever forget, now that you are mine I will treat all of your work orientations as a joke.

As I smiled and headed to work to begin a regular working day, I thought: I couldn't believe that this was already here.

He was my man, and he stood in front of me. I could see him whenever I liked.

The ringing office phone interrupted my sweet thoughts. It was the Director. I did not want to answer, because I had no idea what I would say. I could find no excuse for making the call a few minutes ago. The phone was visible in my corner of the eye.

Now, what do I say? What do I answer you now?

Sophia - Hello, hello Henry.

Henry: Sophia, just wanted to let you know that we're all back together. Aaron is returning to us. Aaron could not stay away for over a year. It was just too difficult for him. You will now be less busy.

Don't listen to it. You must now take revenge for the whole year that he has left you all alone. You can laugh and tell me to have a great day at the office.

Sophia: I know you will pay for everything. So stay calm, you already know me. I laughed. I wished Sophia good luck.

It was a day I'd never forget. Aaron was able to take over the relationship because I wasn't a good leader.

The man, who was very steadfast in his action and did not move from his position, extended his hand and told me:

Aaron - Squeeze my hand

This is what I did. I went to the elevator as if Arnold were inside the building at 11 o'clock. But this time, I didn't feel like spending ten hours with Aaron. So I led him up the stairs.

Aaron was the first place I went when my car wouldn't leave from work. The only clothes I had were the ones I was wearing... I told him to shower, but he refused... I then went to the bedroom to steal his shirt... That's what I planned to do that night.

After I arrived with his shirt and hair half-dry, I would not change the look of his face for anything.

With one breath, he ran to me and grabbed both my hands and arms.

The warmth and protection I felt.

In that embrace, the two souls united, two bodies became a single entity, and all of life came together. I was taken to the skies by his aroma... A flight towards infinity of souls.

The only thing I felt in the room was the beat of my heart.

His arms were around me, and his head resting on my shoulders. We were guided by an indescribable song that we could not describe and never wanted to stop!

His scent is intoxicating. He knew I could not do anything so, as an attempt to compensate for the lost time, he kissed my head and took it in his arms. He was aware that he could remove everything I wore at any time, without me saying a single word.

Aaron's kisses made me realize that the purpose of physical union was to bring two souls together. Kisses were added to enhance that burning feeling inside. If this wasn't enough, then you would go further to try to touch your whole body until you met those two souls.

I could feel his hands on my cheek, and my fears vanished. He smiled, he came close and placed his lips on mine, and we met lips again, but it was different this time, and I felt AAaron's naked body on me. A shiver ran through my entire body as I felt AAaron's naked body. No one was able to control their emotions, and we had reached the best road possible... The road that led us together.

The room was silent, and only two loudly beating hearts could be heard. I could feel his hands tightening my hips. I also felt his thirst as if it was he who had been living in the desert all these years.

He was full of air just above me. The smell of my skin turned you into oxygen. He caressed and touched me with his hands and lips.

There was only our naked bodies on each other.

His sweet words broke the silence, intensifying that moment.

Aaron - With my kisses, I will give your body different positions and shapes. I also want to taste and feel your freshness. Your scent is a medication that I will never stop using. For all of the weeks, days, years and nights I will want you to stay with me forever. Sophia you're mine. Don't leave me ever again. You are my forever love...

His every move was carefully controlled. He never lied, he said I'd feel as if I were in Heaven and he delivered.

Aaron: Please, don't leave me. He cried and placed his head against me.

It was as though I had been born that very moment. My brain was void of all the things around me. Only he was there. It was my duty to soothe him and find out why he cried.

Sophia-Aaron, there's no need to be sad. I cannot see you. My dear, I'm so happy to see you. You seem like an amazing creature to me.

Aaron: I'm in love with you Sophia but have this fear that one day you may leave.

Sophia: Aaron, I think that the emotions we have experienced in recent days may not allow you to fully understand that you are just as happy as me.

Aaron: But Sophia, you've still kept your promise! Aaron - But you still promised me, Sophia!

It was 3:03 am and my cough had disturbed me. I ran to the living area to get something to help calm down. ... It's not working. It was more serious this time than before.

Aaron quickly woke up, and headed to me. When I finally overcame the cough I was having, I went to the bathroom.

Sophia, I'll be with you very soon!

Although I could hear him, I couldn't help him.

While calming myself down, I remembered that I had washed and cleaned my face with a sponge which bled. I didn't think it was important, because I believed that all the coughing could have led to a lession on my throat. yourself.

You looked so exhausted when I opened your bathroom door.

Sophia: I am sorry that you were disturbed in your sleep. Give him the smile that brought him to life.

Aaron's chest was where I found my heart and my cough. This time the cough was gone, but I still couldn't fall asleep!

Aaron woke again when I coughed again on his chest.

What's the matter with Sophia? What's the reason for this frequent coughing? He held out his hand, turned on the lights, then I was very afraid. Then he touched my hair and kissed me, before turning off the light.

The night before, I couldn't sleep. As soon as I closed my eyelids, I felt something squeeze my chest, waking me again. Aaron was informed that I had not been feeling well the night before and would be staying at home. He asked if I had been tired from work. I replied that I did, but understood I needed a rest today. Aaron was shocked by what I said. His eyes were filled with fear. For him to calm down I kissed and hugged him. I laughed and joked, I played with his locks, and I let him know that I was fine. Even though he had tried to hide himself, he left thinking...

The cough stopped for some time after that. After taking some time for myself, I realized that maybe my body was not up to the task. Maybe I was too tired for my body.

Frequently, in the midst of these deep thoughts, my tree, Life, came to mind. I couldn't understand how it could be so close to me. You can believe me when I say that I miss him... but I haven't had the time to find the courage or meet him.

During my time with Aaron I learned a great deal about myself. I imagine I'm still that Arili, with her strong, commanding personality, but now I feel more vulnerable, and I pay more attention. I feel more... Love more... live more!

The same problem is present in our soul in both times of joy and difficulty.

- What if we knew ourselves better?

It was a very long time since I started to understand my feelings, doubts and dilemmas ...!

How do you solve all of this without experiencing it yourself?

After a few months, I felt that it was reasonable to visit my parents not only with them but also with a friend.

My father was going to be very happy. I was filled with joy at the thought of his happiness for me.

A strange feeling took hold of my heart as I walked to the house that I had left behind.

It was to pick up some things I had left at my parents' house. Aaron stopped after I told him to.

The car was open, so I got out and planted my foot firmly on the pavement. I could feel them being unstable. Then I took two steps slowly, raised my head... and a cool breeze from the skies passed through me... my eyes were shut by an incredible force which gave me freshness to my soul.

Aaron was patient and waited for me to return. What I experienced was so intense that I could not describe it. I have apologized for my lack of words.

Sophia: I'm sorry I can't describe what you were talking about.

Without saying a word I rested my chin on the back of the seat, and looked through the window. We continued to drive towards my home.

Aaron always shook me hand when I got out the car. As I climbed the stairs, I saw a vase of green flowers and an attractive tree branch. It was in the vase for several months. From its stem it could be deduced that it was healthy.

The envelope on the doorknob gave me an odd feeling. I did not feel afraid, but I felt sadness. I still didn't know why.

Aaron was busy with the vase, so I sat down on the couch to read the letter. My body slowly fell on top of it as I held the envelope. I remained there until my left arm was holding the envelope to my forehead. I had no strength to stand up. Aaron worried about me, so I read on in tears. I had no desire to finish the letter.

You're taking me with you like that, slowly and gradually... Slowly, you're taking my hand.

It was as though I had met my twin at an early age when I tattooed your arm, but I wasn't right this time!

You should have known everything I was thinking at the time! You should have been told how wonderful Life is and how much joy it brings you. !

Sophia is a woman with an angel's soul. I am in tears. Since I am no longer strong enough to move, I have been waiting for your arrival. Even the stick which helped me up until I met you can't lift me out of this position!

It's the end for me. How much more I can say, but I still wait for you. I want to see you again before I shut my eyes. But maybe you will not come. I planted something in your life that would bring my daughter, Life, into your home, hoping this Life blooms and grows on your heart.

The only thing I'll do is wait to let all the people know who couldn't tell me on that particular day.

"Farewell, Lady of an Angel Soul!"

The person that is well known but did not possess the power to be well-known.

Michael.

The pain of losing him and not having enough time to enjoy his life longer was what made me cry. The letter made it clear that I would not be able to meet Michael again, since the person who sent the letter represented the clinic in which he spent his last few weeks.

From this letter, I could only take away the farewell...and the life branch that had instilled me with fanaticism.

How many lives have we lost that were never lived?

What is the importance of the moment? It is important to be in the moment! You spoke out loud what you were thinking.

The tears in silence can be so thrilling that the skin burns when the tears touch your eye. They are trying to escape from a situation where they lack the energy to remain!

After years of not sitting at the piano I was angry and removed with tears its dusty cover.

Without saying anything, I began to cry and was moved to place my finger on the piano! The tears fell like notes on the keyboard. I did not want to cut my fingernails to clean them away!

It's impossible to live without my father who taught me how to play the piano. She was a great friend to me during those difficult times and I decided to hide her for many years to avoid returning with the emotions I could not handle.

Today I realized that I had to deal with her. I was supposed to have learnt the piano. I shouldn't have closed it because I could have saved myself. Without living, I'd left people behind for years... My most beautiful love was put to the side to hide those feelings that needed to be felt...

As Michael described in his letter.

What to do with such a long day? Aaron and I did not find it easy to drive to my parents.

Sophia Aaron: I would like to visit the tree that has given me a branch today to be with me each day. He deserves my thanks.

Then I began to walk towards her.

I had learned a great deal from the woman who had been silently instructing me for so long, but it was not enough because Michael thought that it would be reasonable to have a piece of her with me each day.

The light breeze that was blowing that day was blowing its leaves to the left and right.

How small I felt beneath her is not something that can be expressed in any other language than the one of my soul. She was magnificent! With my head raised, I saw Life seeming to be even more beautiful. It was as if the world were thanking me.

My whole body was filled with energy and I couldn't take my gaze off of it. With a laugh I'd never done before, I smiled and closed my eyes. Two tears filled up my eyes and sat on my jacket.

When I came up to you I hugged the girl... but my arms couldn't hold her due to her size.

Sophia: Please forgive me, Life!

It was not by accident that I had given that tree the name Life. I always believed that we should live like trees. It was a promise I made to myself and to her to go to Michael, even though I wouldn't get the chance to hear all of his advice.

The steps of the life will be taught to you again - I told myself as I left.

The car had not yet stopped, so I opened the doors, ran to the floor, and then jumped into the arms of your father.

Sophia: "How he missed you, You squeezed him."

Father - You will finally be able smile at your family again - He kissed me on the head and walked to meet Aaron.

As I left, I took my mother's hand and hugged her as tightly as I could. It was important to me to have some time alone with him to tell him all that I'd experienced in this period that I hadn't had the chance to see him.

After our warm conversation, I went into the kitchen, where mom, as usual, had decorated and prepared all her dishes. As I ran towards them, I heard my father speaking to Aaron.

Father - She tried to tell me lies, but she forgot that I knew her better than herself. He laughed while talking with Aaron.

He was telling me about the situation where I asked dad to stop Aaron working at the bank by intervening with some of his friends.

Sophia: Dad, it's time to eat. Don't tell me stories from the past that I can barely remember. I gasped.

Father spoke in a soothing voice, and Aaron, an orator who listened attentively, didn't speak. It's always been my dream to be just like him. I only think that I am like him when it comes to suppressing feelings and keeping quiet... But I was not as mature as he. The right words were said at the right time, and he was a man of wisdom.

This was not a thought I entertained for more than a moment. The thought of being without him for even a moment was not something I wanted to think about.

I had a great weekend with my family and mom made some big changes in her bedroom that really surprised me.

Belle's pictures were archived. There was just one picture in the center of the room. A photo of my father and I playing was taken where we both were laughing. Belle smiled back at me as I approached the photo.

Sophia: Here are my two sisters! This is our best picture. Belles was in my photo and I had pointed her out as though she were in front of me.

I had fallen asleep in Aaron's embrace, as usual. But the cough again woke me. The main thing on my mind was to take care of my dad, so I didn't get out of bed. I just covered my mouth and coughed, while pointing to Aaron to not be alarmed.

The repeated condition did not exhaust me physically or mentally. After my cough had been relieved, I felt a deep sadness in my chest.

The coughing was so bad that I could not sleep and I kept the towel on my hands all night.

The blueness of the day began to dominate the sky as I looked out the window. The towel was bloody again. I could not leave it behind, wash it or hide it. Something told me to go and see my father, as he had begged me for years. The mirror showed me a different face from the previous night, but it was a good thing that the next day was needed. My father wouldn't be helped by my new look, so I decided to return to my house.

Sophia, you came to my mind in my dreams tonight. Dad addressed me very seriously.

Sophia: Well, it's too bad we disturbed your sleeping. I smiled, and I sat down at his feet like I did when I was a child. He looked back at me with a childlike look. The look I gave him made me feel like I was asking him to not worry, or to be stronger than he had been before or that I agreed with him and told him he needed to be concerned ...!

It seemed real to me. This time, I will tell you to stop coughing. He spoke in a tired tone.

The man looked left, right and up as he walked away from the couch.

Sophia: I promise to my dad this time, I will do it. It's going to be the first thing that I do. I asked him for something I didn't need and threw myself in his arms.

Sophia: Please, hug me daddy.

The man put me into his arms, hugged me and assured me that I could always find comfort in these arms.

Aaron repeated to me that he had been so happy to finally meet my family.

Sophia- Aaron: My father was worried when he heard me coughing the night before. I should stop checking. Today, I could feel his anxiety and can't continue.

Aaron had fled from me when he saw the towel that was soiled again. It appeared to me as if I were also telling him that he needed more strength in order to perform the check. I wasn't sure I wanted to do that. Aaron was quiet for a few seconds as I was not speaking to him in his normal voice.

Aaron, are you saying that I too should be concerned?

Sophia: I'm not sure, I'm not familiar with Aaron.

I replied to you by resting my head against the seat of the car, where the only company that I had was the sky.

The cough did not return that evening, and Monday worked as usual. It was not possible to accept any other obligations in the afternoon as I promised to myself and to the tree to go see Michael. So I went.

The next afternoon, I drove to Michael's house where he lived now.

It was only the first time I met him, but I felt he left something in me. Or maybe I gave him too much Michael... What you give in many life situations is more important than anything else.

Aaroni: I get the feeling that you won't be mine. You are searching for feelings that nobody else has ever experienced.

Sophia: I'm going to be with you for the rest of my days. I kissed and smiled at him.

The kisses I had with Aaron were very special. They opened up the whole world for me. There was nothing I could hide. Not even my most secret thoughts about the disappearance of every human being. He was the only one!

Aaron was for me the expression of emotion, love and movement.

The smile I had on my face spoke volumes. This was something I never thought would ever happen to me.

Henry, who was extremely happy about our happiness and work, expressed his satisfaction with Henry's work.

It was at this point that I didn't understand myself. It occurred to me at times to return to the person I used to be... But how distant and gloomy it appeared to be...

While Aaron took a shower I laid down on the sofa and put on some of my favorite songs... I was taken away by a calm, losing touch with reality...

My eyelids were tired and it took me longer than normal to open them. The only thing that blinded my vision was a strong, white light. It was so bright I had to blink and close my eyes. It was different from the bedcover I used every night. Something told me I wasn't at home. I tried getting up, but couldn't.

With the strength that I could muster, I was able to pull myself up from my left hand. I felt that both my mind and conscience were becoming clearer.

The floor was very clear to me. Then I got up, half-lying down. I tossed the white collar onto my chest and pulled it to me as fast as light.

After a few seconds of tightening up my chest, and making a fist on the bed to express my sadness, a sense of calmness came over me. As I tightened the collar on my chest and looked through the window, it was the same feeling. The sky was blue, even though it was minus degrees Celsius outside. As if I was smiling at myself, I smiled up at the blue sky. The calmness I felt was really just a surrendering to the truth that I couldn't hide anymore.

At the beginning, I was already a rival. You know where you want to go, but it takes work and determination to reach there.

It was as if I didn't even think. I am not sure if I blocked them or merely had no need to have any thoughts at all.

The truth can speak to you very loudly at times... It is only right to confront the truth ...!

The voice in the hallway pulled me away from this truth.

Doctor: We must examine the situation. Today, it's not possible to let the woman leave the hospital.

Aaron- She won't be able to sleep without me. I cannot leave her here alone!

His voice was trembling, and it was obvious that he did not believe in what he said. He was aware that I would not be returning home.

Doctor - Her strength is such that medicine can't explain why she was able to stand up in her condition. I ask you to not make it difficult for us and instead to believe in her and in ourselves. The doctor spoke to you in a soothing tone.

Aaron didn't believe me, and his pain echoed throughout the pavilion.

Just now, I found joy and put my hand where I thought I might have an unwanted one. Half standing I put my hands on my thighs and threw down my legs. I then lowered my head without touching the floor and breathed as hard as I could.

It was clear to me that this would my final challenge. I also knew it would be more challenging as I heard a voice in me tell me I wouldn't win!

It sounded like an emergency when I heard quick steps in the hall.

Nursing - Please, Sir, You Can't Enter The Room - A sound of footsteps was heard but the nurse didn't know why.

It was a powerful force which slammed the door against the wall. Aaron was in front of my face.

He rested on my knees, letting all the internal fatigue go. I pressed my lips to the accelerator and thought of how far we'd come to be with Aaron. It wouldn't have been enough to block him even if all staff and doors were closed.

Sophia - Did you come? Well done. I was missing him. I smiled, and I brought his head to my chest.

Aaron: I'm here to bring you home, because I cannot live without you. He said, hoping my illness would disappear with my departure.

Sophia: Neither you or I are aware of this. We must respect the doctor's advice. One thing is for sure, I do not know how much longer I will be unable to come see you. But you are welcome to come stay as many times as you like. You asked him to cool down.

Aaron - Forever!

Sophia - Then listen well, Aaron. Does that answer suffice? - I asked him smiling.

After I received the strength I'd had with me all my life, it became clear that I was the only one who could control the situation. They will have to live without me until the pain is cooled by time. No one can tell you how long. My pain was mysterious, but theirs was certain. I knew I was doomed. To help them, I took the situation into my own hands.

Aaron: Please speak up. You force me to prove you're still there if you refuse to speak.

Sophia: Here I am, and now you will hear my answer. It's like I never stopped. I am feeling great, despite having nothing. I'm a little tired but it doesn't make me love you any less!

The man squeezed my legs and placed his head in my lap. I was so embarrassed to admit that it hurt me.

It's time to speak about my disease, that has been with me for so long, and I never felt it. It was the first time I had ever seen someone enter me, and I wasn't aware of it. He hadn't been invited at all ...!

There are only two options in such situations, and I'm not the only one. You can either become one, travel consciously to the final destination, or find yourself at the end of your disease. Although I hadn't planned my journey in advance, I knew that it was the wrong direction. There was no going back. Why would I want to be led? Why should I be guided?

This disease is something I would like to elaborate on: If you have a fatal disease inside of you, then you do not belong in this world. You have to be very careful not to try and explain it to anyone else.

It is not your fault that it can take over, take your strength and make you hopeless.

You may even lose your identity. You will need help from someone to complete the small tasks of the day. It is only the will to fight that is left, and that is what made me stand for all the people around me.

In such moments, awareness is key. It will help you to succeed and will leave a lasting impression on your family.

You will have an internal war for what you've not lived. You realize that how well you live is more important than how long you have lived. At this stage, it is too late to grasp the truth because death and consciousness are intertwined.

You are often more troubled by one single thought than you are by the actual disease.

Why did I not live without condition? !

Since I've always aspired to set an example for others, I made it my goal to do so myself.

I remember a moment spent with a friend. To prepare for the event, I cut my hair after a certain period. I had long, curly hair that reached my shoulders. My doctors said it was essential. It was psychological to teach myself to have short hair at first, until the thing that no girl can go through is complete hair loss.

Guinthal Sophia Sophia Sophia Sophia wow, why? How did you get all of those hairs out of your heart?

Sophia – Why? What's wrong?

Guinthal: Your hair made all women jealous!

Sophia: They used to exhaust me but, now that they're short, I can spend less time with them.

Guinthal: But now your face is still an angel face.

When we were having this conversation in the bathroom, Guinthal had been a girl that had captured my interest. He lived a life I respected. She was determined, respectful, smiling and always had a good heart.

Guinthal didn't know what I went through but he helped me to understand my appearance in other people's eyes.

You never know what the answer will do to others. You are not you, this is my disease. You are put in a maze that is so complex you can't find your way out. But you must go through. He has "burned me" so many times, yet I've tried to hide it from other people. Even when I did see someone's compassion, it was not something that I wanted to happen.

Many times I've fallen asleep on unforgiving surfaces, knelt in pain and looked to the doctors for help with painful eyes. I also played with veins, trying to get the blood sample that doctors need to diagnose further, or to track the progression of my disease. My hands wanted to go into my lungs, and I was determined to pull this friend out. He had been growing deeper every day. It was often a source of great discomfort for me and funny to those who didn't know the reason why I was so sad, sleeping in the city flowerbeds...

In my mind, we should live in dignity and with respect. My illness has no dignity. It was hers from the moment I could not control myself in her presence...

I've never been happier than when I was in this situation, this condition, this road of no return.

Here's what I would say to someone who has been told that they have an incurable illness.

You don't even feel your body. It's like it's not you. The tears that I shed in those moments were only for my loved ones. Although no one else has ever been in my situation, it was because their souls hurt. It was such a painful experience that I would have liked to reach inside and remove the organs.

It took me a while to realize that I was sharing my body with my spirit.

This made my life more painful, but it also burned away my very existence. This does not occur because we know that we will soon leave this world, it occurs when we leave the people we love, the ones we have sacrificed for, the ones we would give our life for... those who were our oxygen during our life.

It's worse now because I'm even more miserable. I've always believed in supernatural forces, and I'll tell you today that I've asked for the removal of the soul pains after Belle died. I've always preferred physical pains, but I'm not getting them the way I wanted. You will only be able to live with successive pains in a body not yours.

Aaron did not want to leave my side, but I was able to open the door with an ease that I had come to expect.

My father always checked to see if I was asleep or awake when I would fall asleep. Even though my father thought that I was sleeping, I heard the door open. My father would often repeat the same phrase to me when he realized I wasn't asleep.

Have you slept? You will have to wake up very early tomorrow and won't be able to function.

This is how he would open the door to the room I spent a lot time in. Aaron stood up.

Dad took the stance I was familiar with, that of an emotionally strong man, who was trying to hide his feelings in quietness where nobody could see them... But this time, I would not allow it. I got up and I threw Aaron away.

Sophia: Now I'm the one who will play that game. You will never see me without a big smile. You hugged him.

In those moments, I saw the most precious moments in my life spent with my mother and him. The tears poured out of him. Although it was difficult to watch him cry, I understood that it was important to him. It was so bad that my chest began to tremble, I also fell out of his arms.

Father, I just need two minutes to leave. He left after telling me.

The emergency stairs were very near my room, which was located on the third level. I could hear his footsteps going down. The pain in my body was so intense that I went up to the window and hid from the sound of his footsteps. He did not deserve it!

The dancer was dancing in the street. I opened my window a bit to check. My window was ringing with a loud voice. It was a howl which had been going on for many years. The soul of a person who couldn't stand it... I can hear his voice in my heart.

My head was raised and I wanted to shout at the skies why? I knew that I would not find the answer... I laugh when he speaks loudly.

My mother and father did not allow him to visit because I was very sure that he had a serious spiritual condition. He also wanted to verify my state of health himself.

We all have missions in life and I was successful at each one. But this mission, for me, was the hardest. Before and inside myself, I was in a delicate situation.

Sophia: I am listening carefully. Aaron took my hand and closed it, uniting you forever.

Sophia: I have promised to my father but also you. I promise that we'll make it. I only need something from your side.

Aaron: I'll do anything for you. He put me into his strong and warm arms.

Sophia: During the whole ordeal I want only that you love me. That way, you'll become my energy, and I will your energy. It is only this way we can come together. Aaron, I love you. We love you more than ever before.

Aaron: Then I'm sure you can trust me.

The white dress that I was wearing at the hospital with the flowers was removed by him. He removed my white dress with some flowers from the long, thin shelf.

Aaron: I'll try on your clothes now, because it is more convenient to take them off. He pulled me closer to him and smiled.

Aaron, do you know what we're going to be doing now?

Sophia: I could not even understand your thoughts, just as usual.

Aaron: We'll go back home with your dad. Me, your father and you will have dinner as usual. We'll call Mom and have her virtually with us. Tonight, I'll cook dinner for you. The ordinary will become extraordinary. Every day will be unforgettable.

Sophia: That is why I'm in love with your whole being. I smiled at you from my soul when I replied.

Our whole life is spent building walls. A feeling flows that brings us together, not drowns us. We are the only ones, who after years of building walls feel pain. We need to understand that these walls are what has damaged us, not love.

She was there and she tried to find a way for her love to flow, even when she could not...

Love is a Temple... We will return one day. And you'll understand everything... but it will be too late.

It was then that I realized the real meaning of life. I may have been late, or I might not be, but it was never too late.

Aaron, wake up and relax more than ever before. We will be working today, so prepare yourself for a day that will not be like any other.

Sophia: I finally wanted to return to my normal life. You've spoken to your doctors, right? Can I resume my former life now?

Aaron: "Better yet, brighten the lives of everyone today as well." He then kissed and went into my closet.

You will be deciding today!

Sophia: You always made the decisions for me, even though I did not have you physically present. I smiled and curled my arms under the pillows to watch him try to decide what to wear.

After three weeks of not being allowed to be engaged, I thought that everything was over as though I'd dreamed and I returned to my regular life. It wasn't quite like that. Aaron was the one who chose my outfit for that particular day. I knew that this would be Aaron's last day of work.

He didn't tell me where the clothes came from that he wore to work. The dress was a white and black one with a collar on the top and a matching bottom that showed the buttocks and legs. Black jacket to dress and manage the body comfortably. To feel comfortable and in control, I need black shoes with square heels.

He thought about everything. From my clothing to the way I'd get to work and any other details, he had it all planned out.

Aaron was able to tell me that I accepted the reality of my situation and wanted to bring peace to everyone who cared about me.

Henry was opening the door. I read his eyes, even though he smiled and tried to tell me a lie.

Henry: Come and see the mess you've made in our office. Grabging my left hand, he sent me into my office which, from my position, was a mess.

In some of the most delicate times in my life I've had people reach out and send me positive vibes... as if they were telling me we are there with you. My left hand tightened only twice - once at Belle's funeral and again today when Henry died.

The left hand support was shaken with an expression of special emotion.

I will support, guide, and help you... I am in such pain, I do not know what I would do without you.

The gesture I was interpreting by squeezing my left hand is similar to what you have said. Henry also squeezed my hand, and he didn't release it. I felt that he wanted to tell me: "We will have a difficult time without your presence."... My life would be very hard without you for a very long time. We express these feelings and thoughts involuntarily with small, unconscious gestures.

Sophia: Henry, I'll always be there for you. I guarantee that you will be near me. Sophia - Henry, I will always be with you. You'll never leave me.

The glass door opened where I spent the most beautiful time of my life. There were many letters in the office, but all of them were dedications. The dedications were all different, from the most creative to the least. But one stood out above the rest.

Anonymous - In life, I'll work to become like you. It is not possible to be like you. Stay unique!

Aaron was sitting at his desk when I first saw him. He was on her desk today, holding a white wine glass. It was only at that moment, when I was sitting in my chair in the office, did it make me want to sit down.

Aaron was in front of my glass between us, but I opened the door this time and jumped into Aaron's arms.

Aaron, the spiritual beauty I'd ever seen, was beyond compare. His unique personality, his stunning beauty, and the glass of wine he had on the table were all a part of that. I fell in love all over again with Aaron.

Aaron asked me for a couple of minutes on the way home.

Sophia: You go ahead to the car. I'll follow.

Here I was, alone, in the flower garden, where I'd seen people walking around, looking for information or playing chess, children fighting and playing, couples kissing passionately. It was me too. I used to look at you through that window, and never felt the courage to join in this everyday life. The high palace was my home for a long time. I closed my eyes and said goodbye with tears to the place where I had spent a large part of my childhood.

Today, I'm at the second home. This is the house that will carry the burden of this disease to the very end. There is no need to call it by the name we know, because there we feel like we're in a second house, with just one exception: we're naked. Each time I am in his presence, my thoughts stop and an icy feeling envelopes me.

You can't convince yourself to get up and move around to make it on time for your next appointment. The weight inside you is so heavy that it makes the back look like it was carrying its heaviest load ever.

When the automatic door opens again, I am stopped. After taking three steps away from the door that opens automatically, I lift my head to feel the weight of frost which has been suffocating me begin to melt. With my head raised, I carefully examine the entire three-story building. My feelings are warmened by the effort, dedication, care and professionalism shown by the staff.

The smiles are there even when they face physical or spiritual challenges. I was able to speak with more of the staff, and they told me often that the patients have an unfathomable spiritual problem. They are beautiful people!

Sophia, I'm curious to hear how you are feeling in my presence.

Aura: I will show you. Each day, I turn my back to that door and shake all the weight off. You can leave anything for up to eight hours. I can put off my problems for eight hours but not those of patients! Sophia: I'm going to let you in on a little secret. You do more for us than you think! When I leave, I will be leaving my problems for 8 hours outside. All of them have been forgotten.

Here's how we behave. He took my arm and put on the vigona, which delivered the next chemo through my blood.

Many times, I forgot that I had a slow-moving disease. This day I had devoted myself to cooking. I prepared a special meal for Aaron and I. It was a healthy branch of Life and I came to you in order to welcome it. She would also grow, just as Life did. I knew the time would come when we would have to remove her from that apartment. One day, the apartment I gave him wouldn't be big enough. If I wanted to match my mother's time, then I needed to get it planted.

In the living room we had a small table that was used only for documents. Under the lamp shade that was placed on the furniture in the living room, I left the letter my "second family" had sent me.

Stress, feelings, fatigue, chemotherapy... It was not given to me enough time. Today I read the book.

We had three large windows in the living room. One of them was the length of a wall. There I spent quite a bit of time. Before the window I laid a white artificial blanket and sat in front to enjoy the beautiful sky. It was for this reason that I chose to read it there. The color chosen for the letter was the same as the envelope. The pink color was exactly what I like.

They needed A4 size paper to fill out all of that text. It's not clear why I sent the letter back to look for the last paragraph. The farewell words, that I didn't want to read or hear, were not written in the letter. The word "goodbye" was not to be seen. After a quick glance, I realized the letter had been written solely by Henry. He quoted from his co-workers at the end, but it was not what I had thought. Henry wrote me a personal letter.

Henry's Letter

I'll start at the beginning. Today, I would like to say something I never told you. You entered my office that day as a potential candidate to fill the vacant post. It seemed that a presentation with delicate words would be the answer to everything you had said. You were attracted to those curls and held them in your hands for the entire time that you stood before me. You seemed to have a difficult time controlling their moods. You were speaking again when the curling hair fell onto your eyes. This time, your hands were busy with gesticulations, so you blew to get it out.

You said something to me that made my office light up with your smile.

You can tell that I am a great manager. What kind of person would like to be surrounded by caprices "??

Nothing has changed since that day. Each corner of the apartment we use for our activities was lit. You were my point of reference, even though I didn't say it. You can influence anyone who comes close to you with your positivity. Your actions are all unique. You're unique when speaking, unique when deciding, unique even when making a mistake. Your actions have changed us all, and I must admit that you've changed me as well! Your words changed my perspective on life.

It was not my intention to talk about your work. I wanted to learn more about you and the unique world that you live in. This unique world has taught me so much and changed my entire perspective on life. You have been so kind to me that I could not help myself but keep it all for myself.

This time, I fear it'll fade. I feel uncomfortable without you. As you said, I'll try to do it your way.

White and black are the two colors that will always strike us in life. Each has its time! We will sometimes start out with black, then white. This would be ideal, but it is not always the case. Even in white corners, we can overcome black with maturity "!

No conversation with you has escaped my memory. You will be successful in both white and black. In this case the road doesn't matter, but what you do at the end.

You made it, no matter how the ending looks. You succeeded Sophia, we all have a goal and some of us do not succeed.

You will be missed at all times. You will be missed in the office. As an example, we will miss your presence. Your smile is a gift to all of humanity.

For Unique Sophia.

Henry!

It was a very tiring cough. I had to keep going to the bathroom to get rid of it. I found a spot to hide in order to avoid being seen.

The coughing is killing me.

My hands were no longer strong enough to hold the sink. I ran out of energy. The tiles were wrapped around my knees as they buckled. My left hand hit the tiles, I coughed and tears came from my eyes. With my right hand, I squeezed my chest to show:

This is enough, I do not deserve it!

My mind begins to think in a different way when I lie on the floor of the toilet. My strength helped me to face the challenges of life. The door kept slamming, and I couldn't answer Aaron. Aaron was calling me, but I couldn't answer him. The door kept banging.

So I got up by turning to the right. Before the mirror I saw someone I no longer knew. It was exactly as I had predicted. My throat and lips were bleeding. I looked down to the floor. The blood was on the floor, so I cleaned it with a towel. Next, I went to the mirror and cleaned my face, while coughing.

Sophia: Aaron, i'm leaving now. I am fine.

He was leaning on the door and sitting in the hallway.

Aaron: I'll wait for you here. Please don't shut the door. He spoke to me with a loud voice.

He was crying but because his chest was so full he could not help making that bitter sound!

This was actually the moment I realized the situation! Then I opened the door to the bathroom. Aaron jumped up and grabbed me by the waist. He didn't even wait a moment. He was my only refuge. I had no choice but to surrender. I knew I could trust him and felt both stronger and weaker. The corridor never ended, and I was so relaxed in his arms.

Sophia: I'm not going to get up from this position. Please hold me for as long as you can. You tightened around his neck.

Aaron: Together, we can achieve unimaginable feats. Now you can't do it alone.

As always, there was music playing in the living area. Aaron placed his hands on my back and I held my face with my hands. With a kiss our souls were united.

My body was filled with a mix of positive energy, emotions, pain and sadness. Passion and an indescribable feeling of love were also present. The corrected neurons seemed to be in front of me... My legs said no but the speed and adrenaline of the take-off had penetrated me.

He had told me he loved me and would continue to do so. Only he could have known. This moment was deserved.

They called me "The Laughing Man" in my second house.

- Curling in the right spirit.

Even though I had the same illness and was at the same location, I felt lucky because I knew so many other stories. I wanted to relieve the pain. I'd change history. It was much easier to me to be there alone. The next time I had chemotherapy, I would always leave first.

My right foot would be on the small wheels and my left on the floor, while I would press until I was able to move my entire body down the corridor. Pearl was there, and we are going to do chemotherapy today.

Sophia: I'm going to stay here and not move for a while. When it is time to go, they are going to grab me. I laughed, so I tried to make the next chemotherapy easy for her as well.

Her eyes told a different story, and her pain was not the same as mine.

Sophia, Pearl? How are you doing today? It's a stupid question but I need to ask it today. I was surprised to see him looking more exhausted than usual. I wondered what had changed.

Pearl: I am very, very close. He replied, turning his face to the opposite side. I couldn't see him cry.

Sophia: I am also close, like you. I extended my hand in search of her hand.

Pearl: Sophia, this is a delicate situation. And made him cry. The tube that delivered the medicine mixture was blocked. Pearl seemed to be suffering from something more serious than I had imagined.

Sophia: Please tell me otherwise, I'll get up! I- I am signing that I will remove Vigo from my car!

Pearl: Please, don't. Give me some time and I will tell you everything.

In that moment, I felt a sense of anxiety and fear. I asked myself: What if there was something I couldn't help? I then directed my left arm to her and squeezed her. I wanted her to know I cared. As I felt anxiety and fear in those moments, I thought: What if I couldn't help her? It was my duty to do so, whether I liked it or not.

Pearl - I told you about Ajzel.

Sophia: Yes, I know you spoke to me about this beautiful angel.

Pearl - I've said it all now... Pearl - But now I've said everything...

Sophia: You don't think I really understand you.

Pearl: No, this is not as you imagine! He turned his head to let go of the tension in his chest.

Sophia: Then, tell me what it is and what I can do. I swear I'll do it. - Although I was not aware of the details, I made a promise to her. I did so because I knew that something more important was bothering her.

Pearl-Ajzel is suffering from severe heart failure. Only a transplant will save her!

He shifted his entire body to make the position more comfortable. He sat down, looked at the ceiling and began to cry.

It was impossible for me to speak to anyone or anything. As I could feel her pain, I took her position. As I held her hand, tears poured down my cheeks, and we soaked our pillowcases, faces, and hair.

The next day, I was unable to get out of bed and walk alone to the place where Aaron was always waiting for me. Aaron let you come to me and carry me to his car in his arms.

Aaron: Today, they really had an impact on you. He made me laugh like usual when I returned from chemotherapy.

He didn't answer me, but I shook him so hard that my feet wouldn't touch the floor. He was very aware of my situation, but he kept the promise that he made me.

Aaron: Now, tell me. Did you not start out well? Or did you finish badly? He guided me as I drove the car back home.

Sophia: It began as usual and I will finish the same way!

As I held my head up and kept my eyes fixed on the sky that seemed to follow me wherever, Sophia said: "It started as usual. It finishes like it always does!"

Aaron: We hadn't decided in that manner. You have to prove to me that we had already decided on two people traveling this route.

Sophia: I'm missing you, and I don't think I can live without you in my next life! I replied with a glance at him. Like Pearl, I tried to conceal my tears as I stared at the window again.

You can't fall asleep at night. Self-inflicted disease. You can't sleep when your cells are infected ...? It is not the physical state of the body that makes you sleepless, but the mental and spiritual one. You feel like the story will end soon. This was also a sleepless evening. The scarf was thrown over my shoulder and I directed you into the salon. The lamp was on in the hallway, which I turned on. But the rest of our house went dark.

With a smile, I caressed the Life branch. Half-full moons gave the skies a sparkling glow. This time, I sat down at my normal seat and pointed out the window. I also wanted to enjoy the cooling breeze. Closed my eyes and rested my chin on my knees. I let the moonlight take me along. I felt the wind move my hair with such delicacy, it seemed like he was massaging me.

The mind danced with other thoughts. It seems that you can't even find a moment of calm within yourself.

- Will this ever end?

This situation is also getting to me... This situation is also affecting me. It can make even the most strong people weak. My hand was on his shoulder and I said, "I'm sorry." I dropped a tear onto the floor.

When are you going to stop pouring rain uncontrollably?

Aaron: We cannot control the situation, but can alter our perspective. I brushed away the hairs that had fallen into my eyes. He hugged and hugged behind me. It was as though he wanted to assure me that i would be safe there.

The chemical products also eliminated the smell of my skin. The cancer in my lungs was a familiar place. There was no need to move. Although the medication didn't work anymore, it did relieve the pain. In cases of severe pain I would thank them for their support.

Aaron was improving every day. I often wished that you'd tell me that you no longer loved me, as I had a bad attitude. What kind of man would love someone in such a state? It was hard to believe that someone could love me in this condition.

My skin was pale and I was constantly shivering. I wanted to run away. I was afraid he would look me in the eye.

We will realize that there is nothing worse than having thoughts that keep us awake. You get tired! You are embarrassed by them more than your current situation! You are embarrassed just when you thought you had found peace... We try our best to shut off thoughts, but sometimes we fail.

Today, just before I undergo the next chemo, I looked in the mirror. It is difficult to resist the temptation to think about tired thoughts. My mind was completely out of control when I laid down in that bed and gave my arm over to the nursing staff. With my eyes I fixed the sky, just as I do now. Here I want to stop everything. The thoughts had gotten so deep in me, I couldn't even feel my own body. This life seemed cut off to me. The chemical mix that was circulating through my veins felt so cold. It was only then that I could feel a connection between my world and where I wanted to be as quickly as I possibly could.

It's one of those mornings when you just can't get motivated to go anywhere. It's hard to get motivated when you can't find any reason. Benchmark... But nothing works, it doesn't help! You are in a reality that is both bitter and real. Your mind's strength is not strong enough to change it.

Our brain manipulates the situations we face in our daily lives. This force is present in each person and it can be used to make any situation seem like a joke, or a temporary dream. Here's how to deal with life's difficult situations.

Nothing worked. I searched for stimuli to bring out that inner strength. Two tears warmed my side eyes. The room in which I lay seemed to be filled with quick footsteps, but the source was not clear. The people in the room seemed to be so far, yet so near ...!

The hand continued to show special attention for my situation, which caused me even more tears.

Aura: "That's right! Bring out your tears and show me you are still with us!" He said in a soft voice.

Aura and I share a spiritual bond. As I've already mentioned, this connection is very special. She seems to love her job, as even the nurse who assisted me began by asking Aura for help when she saw my state.

Aura: Where are you going without my knowing about your entire special world? He held my hand while talking to me.
After that, my eyes were no longer on the sky.

I turned to my right, and my entire gaze was focused at you. It was difficult to thank him, I could not find the words. But I did give him a grateful look. I smiled at him with two eyes.

Aura: These are the prettiest eyes I've ever seen, and the best gift that he has given me. He said it smiling.

The name Aaron is the only thing that sounds good to me. Aura's voice was the only thing that I could hear, and it took me from the endless space before my eyes to the name Aaron. It seemed like the name Aaron slowly brought me back from my paralysis. The only thing that came to mind was his promise... I could not see or hear anything in the corridor ...! As I lay on the bed I exhaled deeply, releasing some of my negative thoughts.

What is the most difficult thing to say about these feelings? No, it's not true: you are no longer the same person. You don't even have the time to adjust to your new self ...! This is the same thing as being on a plane that offers you new experiences, sights and sounds every moment... A new spiritual state... But unlike a flight where you get a rainbow show inside, the journey that I am taking is not happy, but it's endless!

I was not able to find the strength in me and stand up because of nausea and fatigue from chemotherapy. He wants to take Vigo out of his veins. It seems that he is the one who caused this situation.

The void in me was overwhelming. I felt lonely and tired. It seemed that the bed itself had taken on the form of an U-J.

Aaron: Now, get up. I'll show you what to do. Aaron finally spoke. He approached, caressing my body as though to rehab me.

The ice that I felt in my heart melted away when he touched me.

I was able to speak before I realized that I had heard him, but I still smiled with a smile that is not interpreted. It's as if the whole face changes shape and sparkles. You only smile when you are saved.

Light moved from my heart to my face and arms. When he stood next to me, the blood flowed at a faster rate.

Aura: I have finished today's cycle. Lord, please give me the correct time. Aaron was pointed out with an expression full of codes.

Aaron - Thank you, Madam.

Aura: You made my day today. He kissed me on my forehead to encourage me.

Aaron: "Listen, if the kiss she gives you brings your smile back to life, then I'll be jealous." He laughed and placed his lips against mine.

Sophia: I'm very tired. I was so choked up that I didn't even know how I managed to speak.

Aaron: That's why I am here. He placed his hands underneath the blanket that was covering my body, and began massaging it. His hands passed over my shoulders as he massaged my back. Then I turned my head to the left and handed his hands, which looked just like the hands of an accomplished pianist.

There was no sleep as the night fell. To defeat my thoughts, I would lie down in bed. They caused me as much pain as the illness itself. Aaron would grab my hand every time I rotated to let me know he wasn't sleeping. Let go of Aaron's hand and let him know that I would be getting up. He shouldn't try to follow me. Without turning on the lights in the home, I walked you quickly to the living area. The only light I had was that of the hope the darkness gave me. I followed the furniture with my hand and ran my fingers over it as though this were the last contact I'd have with them.

Aaroni had placed my piano at a corner in the living room. This light of hope shone directly on my piano. The twinkle in my eyes made me think I had found salvation. You were touched delicately as I walked up to you. My right hand wanted to play notes as soon as I opened the piano.

It was hard to keep my hands still on the keyboard, even though I had no idea what time it is. Then I put my head and left hand together on the keyboard and started playing with my right. I was completely immersed in the music and forgot about everything for a while. I played as if it were the first time I'd ever touched the instrument.

Hands and mind were in sync, soul and heart flew into a place without title, name or identity, an unknown space. My eyes began to water. Close my eyes, and I'll play the piano with my head raised. The light that was shining in my window made me open my eyes, but I didn't stop playing my piano.

People who understood the purpose of this music, at such an late hour, sat on the railing. They didn't expect me to stop playing, and I knew that. I continued to do so with the same spirit I had felt outside of my window. Then another light appeared, then another, and so on.

I saw several people at once. For the very first time I had spectators that wanted me to continue playing the piano. As I played, it was as though I were presenting my artwork. I would look up and see the windows full of people with lights. I'd smile between the tears.

This moment ends with applause.

Without saying a word, I pointed at the window and bowed my head to say thank you. Aaron kissed me on the neck and hugged from behind.

Aaron, I love you to infinity. We both understand that this is not the life of infinity.

You change so much that you often don't give your life any meaning. As I slowly walked through the hallway of the cancer ward with my stand, I pulled it as though it was my best friend... In the rooms I would smile and greet those who had barely opened their eyelids to see me. This corridor was so long for me ...! What did they think of these walls and how much have they heard them? I often wondered. I often wondered.

Everyone knew me. Some of the doors were shut and others were only half-opened. Even they now knew that Sophia opened doors without knocking. The last door in the pavilion was right next to the window of the corridor. I tried to focus my attention on it. Marisa had moved in temporarily. She was a mother with two grown-up children.

Sophia: How is everyone today? I asked the woman in front of me, sitting right next to her, how she was feeling. He seemed to be more lethargic and tired today than ever before.

Marisa-Mednova was not my child, and I must see you because this could be your last visit. She squeezed my hand as hard as she could, her strength a gentle caress.

It was all her heart wanted in that moment. He was unable to push the button on his emergency bell, which he held in his hand. The stand was used to support my head as I kissed his forehead.

Marisa: Sophia, I've never met anyone so void. He said it when he saw that I was leaving.

The tears filled my eyes, but I did not want her to know that I wept for her, as I felt the same way. As I leaned my head against the railing and directed you towards the window, I was taking care of Vigo, which is the link between the blood mixture with the medication. When I heard Marisa running to her room, my tears began to fall on the railing. They were moving, but I thought they didn't move. My body was frozen. I asked them to help her rehab her as long as her children were with her. My eyes would look at the door to the pavilion from time-to-time, but I was only searching for her kids. Two stars who had lost their twinkle ran towards Marise's room. The handle on the door was all I could see until I noticed the trembling hands that were lowering the handle, and calling out to her mother.

We are here, Mom!

Then I pulled the tripod out with a defiant glance and pointed you in the direction of the room. I laid on my bed and thought to myself,

Here's how to make an unrestrained soul smile today!

What about my mother? What about my dad ...?? Who will be your ally? I was agitated by the unanswered question. All becomes a question. We are all called Mister. It is all a mysterious world. I had so many questions that my own name was a mystery.

Why was Sophia my name? What was the reason I needed a name in order to survive a life where an illness took away your Name, which you believed belonged to you? Why did I get born? Why did I get educated? Why did I make all these sacrifices? Why was my sister taken so soon? Why was my family put through so much?

Why? Why? Why...?

Aaron - Are you thinking? We don't even have the time to think, because we need to leave. Aaron always pulled me from thoughts which took away what I was left with.

Sophia: We will go out when I feel better, my love. You were directing me to the bathroom, and I was to look in the mirror.

Mirror shows the past, and present. Half of the past had still hair, but the present is losing its...

When you can't recognise two people standing in front of your face. Even tears flowed from only the left eye where the hair was. To get to know my new self, I started to pull my hair out of my scalp. Sophia was in front of me with a new face. The look I saw could have broken my eye. The hospital shirt was removed and I turned my back to the mirror in order to reveal the full Sophia.

The kneecaps looked so bare, and the bones were so ragged that I thought they could be ripped off by my fingers. The end without hope.

It's you, Sophia, today. You said to yourself with a convincing voice.

Aaron was standing in the doorway of the bathroom when I opened it.

Sophia: I am Sophia the New, my brand new self, with my all-new look. My strength was taken away by a cry and I could no longer hold my head. My head was not strong enough to hold my tears, so I placed my hands over my face.

Aaron, you are the most gorgeous dog I've ever seen. I believe I love you even more. He wrapped my hands around his neck and took me into his arms.

His delicacy was so strong that I could even feel it in my soul. He placed me on the mattress.

Aaron: I assure you, this is going to be your most memorable day. Just wait. He covered me with the hospital shirt and told me:

Aaron: Promise me you won't think negatively until I return. Resting his lips against mine.

Sophia: It is impossible for me to refuse your request. I smiled at him and he loved it.

Aaron, who was out of breath due to the frantic rush, turned in a blink. He stopped and took out the blue dress that seemed to have a special glow. He placed the dress on a chair and took me into his arms. Then he carefully lifted me out of bed. Together, we took you to the bathroom. The machine I used to take my hair out was so fast that I didn't have time to check where it had taken it.

Aaron: I do not want you in despair, or to weep. You can close your eyes.

With his instruction, my new face started to take over the old one.

Aaron - Open your eyes.

With his hands he took my both hands.

I then explored all of the scalp without finding a single hair. He placed his head on my shoulder, and lightly kissed the neck. With one quick movement, he brought the left hand he had hidden behind his back to his face and revealed the wig.

Sophia, finally straight hair. I smiled.

They are positioned in my mind as though they were the favorite artwork of his. I corrected the delicacy and skill of his hands. As always, I could not read his emotions when I looked into his eyes. He was very good at concealing his feelings...

Then he put me down on the bed and took off the dress. I then helped him to put it on. I wore a black jacket over my shoulders, and the scarf would cover my lower legs. Aaron also took the wheelchair to help me follow in Aaron's steps, as I could no longer walk for long.

Aaron was looking at me and I thanked him. I thought young Sophia didn't look so bad. I was distracted by his presence and didn't think much about my transformation. You have to accept the new body even if it does not make any sense.

It was the first time I had ever been on a road trip. I did not know what we were doing, but I trusted his words. He promised that it would be a beautiful day.

And, I knew that would happen. After seeing the vase containing the Life branch, I was surprised.

Sophia: Why are we in this together, dearest? It isn't a good place for her.

Aaron: Today, she'll take her life! He grabbed me by the throat with wet, protective hands.

Sophia: Then, I will not ask any questions till the end of today. I laughed while kissing my hand.

He would often ask me on the way if I felt well. As usual, I rested my head on the seat of the car and focused my eyes only on the sky. For a few seconds, I held his hand to make sure that I was okay. I was experiencing different emotions. I felt like I had a mix of emotions. I wanted both to laugh and cry. I felt happy, but also sad. In my head, the clouds represented the notes on the piano and the sky itself was the piano. It was a journey I didn't know how long would be, but I wanted to continue it.

The view was so breathtaking that it took even my last breath. My mind helped me get out of the vehicle, despite the fact that I wasn't as strong physically as I once was. The hand I was familiar with squeezed my elbow and prevented me from getting out of the vehicle in an accident that could have caused serious injury.

The hand I could never help! This hand, I couldn't help. He threw himself into my arms with all the delicacy and strength he could muster in his heart. I hugged him as hard as I could, but I had no more strength.

Sophia: You're a treasure to me, Daddy. Resting your head against his shoulder, you said.

AAaron removed the stroller from the vehicle and my dad sat there. My mother was approaching us and I focused my whole attention on her. As I was about to stand up, I realized that I would not be able run. I grabbed the wheel of the chair and began to move until my mother fell onto my lap. I stroked the hair of my mother and allowed her to rest on my lap. Today I needed to prove myself more powerful than anyone else.

Sophia, Queen of my Heart - you said holding your hand out. Will you come with me? Give her a smile to calm her down.

Aaron - This is something I did not expect. It's the best day of my entire life. I was in a rush to say something to play the part that has always characterized my life. I was trying to give my parents the best possible feeling.

During lunch, I often lost control.

As I watched them, I was aware of my own feelings, but wondered how they were feeling at that moment. I saw a large, warm hand that showed signs of age.

Father: Now let's dance like you learned to do when you were a child. He took me into the middle of the restaurant where there was a dance floor.

Sophia: With pleasure, my love.

We both knew that there was not much time, and we needed to get everything out to the other.

My father, I've often felt that my life was unfair but now I must admit I am lucky. My daughter is the kind of girl that anyone would love to have.

Sophia: Dad, this is the moment when we cannot lie to ourselves. You and I wouldn't want to dance this way. You would have loved to dance this way on my wedding. You would have also liked to be around your nieces and nephews. You probably wanted me to dance with you and be joyful every time... I may have also wanted this, but I denied myself. I lean on your shoulder to listen to the heartbeat, which seemed not be inside the chest.

What will happen if I ever find another girl as beautiful as you? He placed his hand on the wig.

Sophia: You can see that your hand is no longer lost in my locks. You tried to make it a special moment for him.

You'll have to adjust to it. I used to lose my fingers through your hair my whole life.

Sophia: Dad, you have to hear it. I donated the organs.

His body was immediately reattached. For a brief moment, his arm detached itself from my hair but then he firmly held it. My throat began to tremble as I exhaled a long and exhausted breath. I replied with a hoarse tone.

Father - I accept and understand your decision. You are a man who was born never to leave.

He placed his head against mine. If I hadn't had the wig on, I was sure that my hair would have been soaked from his tears. But I could not add more words.

Sophia: Dad, you will always have my love.

Aaron, not knowing the cause of my father's tears, began to walk towards us. He took me out of my father's arms, and then we left together. A small pit had been dug by the restaurant's staff.

It was a strange feeling to be in front of a thing I didn't understand, yet it made me feel clean and peaceful. Aaron was coming towards me with a branch of Life. I was directed by the staff, who gave me a small tool to plant the Branch of Life.

Manager: We've decided to put a branch from your favourite tree here. We decided with you and your family to name you Sophia. If you are willing to trust us to take care of the future Sophia tree, all you need to do is to plant it yourself.

Sophia: I completely agree with what you said. I'm smiling.

This moment was frozen in a photo to be cherished forever. In that picture, with that dress in the cart and my family around me as well as a staff that allowed me to take part in this moment I could not help but smile. Branch of Life will live and grow and provide shelter for birds and humans who are near it. My smile may have lit up my face, but I thought that wig was really pretty. Aaron is the subject of my gaze.

Sophia: I'd like to spend some time alone. Aaron and my family are the people I told you about.

I felt detached from the landscape in front of me.

In my present situation I have the same sensation, that is to say, neither feeling like a part of one world or another. The two berries were resting on my knees as I admired the scenery.

In this moment, I am filled with spiritual peace. I instinctively feel the urge to ask God to send it to Aaron and my parents. I covered my face with my hands and my despair rose. This truth was what I sought, this assurance... They didn't deserve any suffering!

I could not stop asking myself a million questions. There were no answers. All of us have a life mission, but we do not know if we have fulfilled it.

What am I? What have you given to life? What would I give you? And what might I do differently?

When you must face your own truth!

To avoid being hurt you have to be willing to hurt yourself. Are we willing to harm ourselves in order to avoid hurting others? It is the way I've always behaved.

I would have been better off living a life of freedom. I shouldn't have been influenced at all. I should have been more aware of myself. You should have been loved more by me.

This is exactly what you see. We make the same mistakes again, despite all of the people in history who made us free. Time is wasted on situations we don't need. No one returns the time we give, and it is our most valuable gene. It's not too late to devote the time you have to good things, to people who deserve it, and to those that need it. In my case it was my lungs. No matter how much I want to control and convince him, it is impossible.

The journey of life is one with you. My journey has come to an end, as I can see in the sky that is reflected before me. The sky won't change, but the birds may fly in different directions, or the shape and color of the trees, clouds, and sun. The sky will be infinite again, the sun will shine as always even though it is often hidden. I'll never change anything.

Cancer had taken over my life. I was left with nothing. I only controlled my eyesight. Everything else fell under its control. His influence extends to feelings, thoughts and everything that is a part of a person. When I look at my hands and open my palm, I am amazed by the transformation. It was very common for me to rub my right with my left, or my right with my other hand. In a normal world, this would be very mundane, but it gave me courage. With that gesture, I could feel the world's hands. As my cough got worse, I'd clasp my hands together tightly and stare up into the sky.

The sky has often been asked if I am in pain because of my eyes. Even the sky would think that this is not possible!

Yesterday ...? However, I wasn't able to. The sky did not perceive us. We can't understand each other. He may also want to speak to us. To thank him for hearing my words and maybe feeling my pain, I turned them into piano music.

Michael said that all I had left of us was our past. Every person who has crossed my path on this trip is a symbol of destiny. Michael was a person you knew immediately. No matter what the situation, we must listen to our instinct. It is important to not stop instinct, but rather give it two legs so it can go wherever it wishes. We will leave behind nothing, except a memorial for those who miss us. Maybe we'll be right next to them in the same direction.

Then I laugh at my idols. Maybe I do need some talent to play the piano I love so much. But I also think that it would be better if it was not locked away for another few years.

When I think of Belle, tears can't stop falling. It is common to add up her and my ages in order to convince yourself that my parents were happy for many years. The bitter years have already passed, but the bed on which I lie makes me realize that they will last longer.

I've never felt bitter about life even in my current state. But there were moments when it was difficult to not ask.

Why?

As always, the nurse who was on duty at the hospital where I had been laid up arrived on time. She opened the window, and as the wind blew outside, the melody of a violin came through.

Sophia: Will you get me up from this bed? I'd like to see this violinist and listen to it. !

Margareth: It may be difficult. The cough could increase. I need to consult the doctor.

Sophia: Why are you trying to protect my health? Don't die today?! If I don't get out, I will die tomorrow... I am dead nonetheless! Take me outside, I'd love to hear and see that violin.

Margareth: I must follow orders. I'll try to persuade the doctor.

The doctor opened the door and gave me a look that met my gaze. It seemed as though it was never going to return, as if that villa would not emit those beautiful sounds that I have ever heard. When the door opened, the doctor took a moment to look at me and then continued. Just by looking at you, I asked that I get out of bed.

We both knew that this bed was soon going to be vacant or that someone would take up the bed in its last days.

Doctor - Sophia can come out. He closed the door and left.

It was obvious that the man felt bad for me. I also knew I looked terrible, and I could imagine that his eyes would be filled with pain. But I did not care. I wanted to see who had played this violin so well, whose hands were producing that wonderful sound within me.

As soon as the gate to the hospital was opened, I immediately felt cold. Or maybe my body temperature could not be matched with the ambient outside temperature. With a look that was searching and a breath of air that ran from me, in that carriage I desperately wanted to find the hands who made those sounds.

A middle-aged male with white hair, a beard and glasses was standing in front of me. He was playing the violin while his eyes were closed. Not only was I in front of the man, but also the only person in a wheel chair. While he was playing the violin I couldn't help but clap. This made him look up for a little while. His hands reached me without stopping as our eyes crossed.

Street violinist: Thank you very much for being here. You are one of the most beautiful girls in the world. I play the violin in front of me, but without ever opening my eyes.

The notes he played with the violin were the only thing that could have brought joy to my face.

What do you call a street violinist? Giving me a pitying look

Sophia: Now, I'm not called by anyone, but you can give me Sophia as a nickname during a conversation. What do people call you? "What do they call you, Sir?" I smiled and asked.

Alan, the hopeless street violinist!

Sophia: Why are you calling yourself hopeless? I looked at him very seriously.

Alan – I play violin every weekend for my daughter without any hope of ever seeing her again.

Sophia: Sir, as I speak to you I could even catch a cold that would eventually lead me to my death. Possibly, as soon as my head hits the pillow I'll breathe my last breath! Sleeping at night may take me slowly... It's possible that I won't be around for some time... but I wouldn't say I am hopeless.

Alan: I'm sorry, but I shouldn't have placed the order in that situation. He was sitting next to me.

Sophia: You do not have to apologize at all to me. You need to move if you want to let your daughter rest. You should visit the center of your city every weekend. You will make many people happy, as you did for me today. You will not be able get out of the situation if you continue to play your violin. Nobody can go back in time.

Are you sure that your daughter will be pleased to see herself in such a state? You think you can return your son to you in this manner?

You will only see girls with wigs on their heads in this place, as we wait for that day when the skies open. This is not what your daughter wants. I ran up to him, shook hands with him.

Alan - Is it true that you said I could go outside? "He answered me while he was sitting near my knees.

Sophia: How will you ever know without trying?

Alan: You're a special person - He told me with a look of surprise.

Sophia: What's the name of your daughter?

Alan: Layla. Layla is their name. Alan - Layla, their name was.

Sophia is what they call her. But, she's still called Layla. I'll greet him. I swear I'll greet him. She will hear her father playing his violin right in the middle the city.

Alan, too, was a strong meeting. As I said, everyone I've met has been for an important reason.

This pavilion is filled with a silence that I find murderous. She didn't like it. I still go to work every day, even though I cannot get up by myself. You can greet everyone and start a short conversation with each person. Many times, I can't answer them, but we still shake hands.

Every day, in this pavilion, I wonder how such pain, physical and spiritual does not create noise but that the peace inside is deadly.

While I was here I watched rooms get cleaned. Every time the staff was cleaning rooms, I would stop in front of it. Everything on the bed was thrown into unwashed baskets. The nightstands and all the contents were emptied in the garbage can. It was now ready for me. The mattresses had been laid out and the nightstands disinfected. A bottle of water was also placed there. Since I've been coming here for years, and I now work 24 hours per day in this hotel, I know that these rooms are rarely empty.

Sophia: Why don't you allow me to enter and say hi? I told you about the nurse pushing my wheelchair when I went to see my friends in the pavilion.

Dany: Because Sophia is a brand new patient who has entered the clinic and doesn't seem to be worried. He told me that pushing the door was difficult and I might have to do it for the first.

Sophia: Okay, then send me to that place, I will knock.

Sophia - Maybe tomorrow.

She was aware that I had achieved my goal, but I could not leave the bed on my own. No one wanted to "disturb" someone who made it clear that he didn't want me to be worried.

Now we have to lay down.

Sophia: Send me into the room. But to be honest, I do not want to lay down. I would rather sit in the wheel chair. I replied to you in a hoarse tone.

In the meantime, he left the door open half and rang the bell. He invited me to call it in the event of an emergency. As soon as Dany had left, I began massaging and rubbing my hands together. My foot was used to try and remove the fuse from the cart that had me isolated in the same spot. My hands were in shape after removing the fuse.

With my hands I began to push the wheel, and it smashed into place. I was able to escape the room with my strength. The wheels were pushed as quickly as I could to reach the room where no one was allowed in. Because I was too fast and didn't have the strength to stop in time, the door opened and Zoterine was woken up.

Dany was coming towards me, after I heard the sound I made when I hit the door to the Master's bedroom. I made a sad look, thinking that Master was going to take me away and Dany lay me back in the bed.

Dany, Sophia, please, don't bother patients in this way!

Sophia, I still have not asked Dany dear whether he was worried by my presence. I smiled to him so I could ask Zoterina about her welcome.

Zoterina: I'm sorry, I wasn't sure. But the girl is welcome to stay. He replied with a sad expression.

Please call me after you finish. He put the alarm on my wrist and directed me.

Sophia: Dany, thank you. I replied to you with a smile.

This was the first pavilion where I did not know what to do in front of this gentleman.

I stood up and went back to my old Sophia, the one with the formal manners.

Sophia - Hi, I'm Sophia. Please accept my apology for disturbing you. Thank you. What's your name? I extended my hand in greeting to him and asked, "What is your name?"

Brian, they call me Brian for a short time. It didn't disturb me and I was not sleeping. Sleeping here is not possible. Then slowly got out of bed in semi-lying.

Sophia: That is how everyone here calls me, and they have for some time.

Brian - what did you do to my bedroom?

Sophia: The reason I came to your bedroom is quite long, if you ask me. Is that good enough? I smiled at you to keep the conversation friendly.

Brian: But we're not girls.

Sophia: I don't know anyone in this group, but it hasn't prevented me from getting acquainted with everyone.

Brian: There is no room for friendship. Today you are here and tomorrow you will be gone. I have no hope for you. You've got your whole life in front of you.

Sophia: How do we live when I am in a wheel chair and can't stand on my feet, Lord? I removed the wig that I wore on my head to answer you.

Brian, I'm sorry. He spoke to me and moved from his bed instinctively. I can see that my gesture was shocking.

Sophia: I don't want to be sorry, but I do need you to assure me that you will allow me to visit as many times as I like.

Brian: Of course you are welcome to come back as many times as you like. You were correct, it is possible to have time for friends.

Sophia: Hooray! I have a new best friend in my life. I raised my arms as if to celebrate.

Brian, can I ask you a question?

Sophia: Here, we can ask whatever, and it will remain here. I smiled at you when I replied.

Brian, how long have you lived here? Why are you so young here?

Sophia: I've got enough time to get to know all the beautiful people on this planet, and I still don't know why. There is cancer in both my lungs, and I don't know how to cure it. The real reason for all of this, however, is still a mystery to me.

Brian: You are a very special person. He was in tears when he addressed me.

Sophia: Do you have children?

Brian - My sadness is due to my family. My daughter is now 37. I've worked my whole life for her. I couldn't do the things a dad should for a daughter. - I asked him, and he replied with his tears streaming down.

Sophia: Eh, fathers are special. He thinks the same way about my father, that he hasn't done anything for me. I have the most beautiful and expensive genes of all; his love. When you look after us, you don't realize how much money you are donating! In this condition, I realize that today he gave me his most beautiful gift. Love and care. You know that nothing is worth anything. You don't realize how much we miss you when you're not around. Even in my next life, I'll need to be led and guided by my father.

Brian, who knows what your family will think of you when they see it?

Sophia: I wonder what he'll do without you? I dropped my head to the floor and hit the alarm. I did not want to weep in front of him, because I knew his pain. I felt as if I caused my father to suffer.

Dany pushed me gently and I asked before I left the room.

Sophia: Can you please come back tomorrow? I believe we still have much to discuss.

Brian: You are welcome to come Sophia as many times as you like. He replied to me, and then greeted with his right hand.

You've managed to melt the heart of a man who was frozen. He said with pride.

Sophia: Dany, You don't get me. If I weren't with Zoterine I would not have been able to fall asleep for those few moments that I did.

Dany-Sophia, take good care of yourself. You can do it. It's hard to believe that I might have to contact the hygienists for the room one day. He made me feel better by placing me in the bed I did not want.

Sophia: You are well aware that I cannot make it. I shook hands with him and smiled, then threw his wig onto the dresser.

Aaron was able to wake me from my deep sleep, which I had fallen into due to the fatigue that this cancer has caused. Now I grab my wig instead of reaching for the table beside the bed to silence the alarm. Only then could I get ready.

I carefully put the wig on. Every day, he used to put me in the stroller with him and we would go for a walk.

Aaron - I sometimes wonder how long you'll stay in this place.

Sophia: What is wrong? What's wrong here? I smiled and turned my head to answer.

Never did I agree to use the elevator down to the hospital yard. As I was leaving, I greeted and looked at everyone. The doctors and nurses greeted me with their hands.

It opened, but I once more looked up at doctors, nurses and other passersby, who had stopped to greet me as I approached the exit. They knew I was there, so the doctors, nurses, and other hospital employees stopped to greet me and let me go. Visitors or passers-by would give me an apologetic look, nod and greet me. All I had to offer everyone, whether they were friends or strangers, was a simple smile.

Sophia: "Look up there" - You said to Aaron, while pointing at the roof of the building.

Aaron - It looks high from here, but...

Sophia: We know it will not look as high from here when we arrive.

The people who were in charge of our case did not take kindly to being convinced. For this very reason, we needed to have a security member accompany us.

Sportswoman, ladies. We must accompany you to ensure your safety.

Sophia: I understand, but I would like a stranger with us. I'll make a friend today. Your conditions are different from mine. I continued to smile as usual.

Sportswoman – This girl is extraordinary. She spoke to Aaron at a very low volume so I would not hear her.

Even though I watched and listened to everything, I couldn't understand why people would say such things about me so often!

A gentleman was with us and he had a special name. It was a name I'd never heard before and it took me a while to ask him.

Sophia: What an interesting name! Ertas is a name I've never heard.

Ertas is a name combination that produces this exact result.

Sophia: Then, it's a combination of two souls that have given birth to a creature special with a unique name.

Ertas - Thank you, Madam.

Sophia: You may call me Sophia, as we are already acquainted.

Ertas doesn't allow Aaron to drive the cart.

Ertas: Sir, please keep her balance. You can give her a handshake and go slowly up.

It's the way I made everyone feel comfortable when they spoke to me. It took longer to ascend, but I wasn't acting differently, and I also didn't use an elevator.

Ertas opened up the door and pushed my cart. I found myself at a height which was indescribable. Aaron helped me to get up close and I gave him an overview of the building.

Sophia, I have something important to say. Please climb the highest point in front of yourself whenever you are looking down. You will only be able to express your emotions after experiencing both sides.

As I sat with my hands on a protective railing that resembled a window, I studied every move and detail. The same thing is happening in every category, but they do it differently. People would be speeding even if I was at the top of a tall building. People rush to get to the office, be at a meeting on time, or to the station of the public transportation. Cafes are full.

Some people with their friends, others alone. Some look up at the sky, while some stare at the crowd in front. The same things are happening from this place, but the only difference is that the dogs in the crowd look for ways to get back to the center of the city to join the other people with their different goals.

The past is not a part of me. I've never known who I am. Had I surrendered in the past to you, I wouldn't have known anyone else I encountered on this journey. You are only confused because you live only in the moment, despite the fact that it is clear that the future does not exist. The sky is above us all, and it gives everyone hope for the future.

Although my cough made this moment a disaster, I did not want to go. It was difficult to speak when the cough started. Aaron was able to understand my request by shaking his hand and making signs. Ertas started to walk towards me but I quickly made it clear that I did not want him to take me away from the spot. The handkerchief I carry with me was placed on my lips and I allowed the cough to go as it pleased. It bled. I handed you my cart and all of my pain.

Aaron: We must go. "He said as he pulled me from the carriage and took me into his arms.

Aaron was holding me, so I did not use the lift. You could see it in their faces. Aaron was a man of piety, and I saw it in his face.

In his eyes, I could never see that I looked bad. He laid me down on my bed and started to take off my wig.

Sophia: "Don't remove it" - Although I'm not sure if I understood, I'm certain that his gesture made him realize that I was determined to keep my wig.

Aaron: I was going to place my hand directly on your head, but the wig would have made it difficult for me to do so. He said, holding his hand down to my face.

He cut off my entire face and neck with the back of his index finger on the right. My hand was so delicate that it could have hurt me with just a gentle touch. His left hand was on my chest, as if trying to ease any discomfort. My chest felt warmer when I threw my arm on his. He threw his hand on mine because it was cold.

Sophia: You have the best feeling in the world of love Aaron. With the last of my voice, I spoke.

Aaron, I love you and will until we see each other again. Then we'll pick up right where the last conversation ended. And rest his lips against mine.

Aaron was strong during this time, and thanks to his strength, I even managed to laugh at myself, and turn anything into humor.

Aaron was very strong during this period, and because of his strength I managed to make myself laugh and to turn everything into humor... We both knew there was no hope.

My vision began to slow down as the cough took over. Aaron was still holding me, but I turned to look at him. Even breathing was impossible. AAaron used an alarm. Everything around me was moving away. Not even the oxygen from the equipment that was on my body affected me.

He was coughing so hard that his eyes turned red. My lip was warm and the liquid flowed along with my neck's heat. My right hand was the only thing that moved. I touched my lips with my palm and pointed my finger in front of me. My hand was red. I held both my hands together on my chest, using the last of the strength in me, and tried to rub it a bit. My vision faded and I could not see anyone in front of me. The hot blood that did not cease did nothing to awaken my cells. Aaron's crying was the very last thing that I carried with me when my final departure from this world came!

Everywhere I heard a strange noise inside that building

Sophia died!

The emergency staircase was flooded with doctors and nurses. No one thought Aril would finally leave. Everyone was eager to contribute.

It was a full room and there were many people in the corridor. In a short time, I halted everything. The doctors left with heads down and the nurses had only tears. Maybe the patients who lost hope are those I helped every day. Even from the top, for a short time, it seemed that all life had stopped in that building.

Dad gasped and grabbed Mom's hand as he walked toward me. In the past few days I kept them at a distance. I did not want my final moments to be etched in their minds. It was not fair, and I tried to protect them from anything that might worsen their suffering.

The face of my father in front me had a new color. It was now yellow and black. Not even the blood was flowing on his face. He was staring at my face. My mother slid her right hand across my forehead as I released my mother's left hand. She rested it on my hands.

"Open your eyes Eli! Get up for your Father!" He told me, kissing my forehead lightly.

She was sobbing and holding her head as she rested on the legs of my body.

Aaron: I'd like you all to be spared this agony.

You only got Sophia?

In that corridor, the father sat with a small handkerchief that he was using as a plaything because it could not remove his tears. My father, who was tall and heavy like me, was sitting in that chair. He looked like a child crying. The man moved his coat, raised and lowered his eyes. The tears on his hands and his hands were trembling.

My father addressed me as Sir. Brian was the man, and my father did not even recognize him. I still thanked him in my head. Brian moved closer to the father until he sat next to him.

Brian: Sir, you are the best person to understand me, because I have met your daughter. She was special, and I had never met a girl quite like her. Therefore, I can understand your pain. You should also be proud of your daughter. It will remain forever! People will probably respect that I'm the first to come up and tell you about this pain. But we think you'll soon realize what an amazing girl you raised. Arilin will never be forgotten and I am sure that something special is going to happen.

Dad couldn't answer but gave him an appreciative look.

My father rested his hand on the shoulder of my mother.

My condolences to you, sir. As you can tell, this is not an ordinary day in the hospital. My mouth was about to say two words I have never said in my career.

Who amongst us wouldn't want to be in her family? Your daughter is the most beautiful girl that I've ever seen as a client. You only meet a person as exceptional as your daughter once, if you ask me. Although I wasn't lucky enough to become a member of her family I still had the good fortune to spend time with her. "Said the doctor, who has been following me through this time.

Aura: Sir, please accept my sincere condolences. I apologize for my inability to contain my feelings. Aura extended his hand to you and directed you towards the father.

Father - I'm grateful, please don't apologise, no one can control me today. Your father replied, squeezing his hand.

Aura: I'm sorry, I don't know the best time to tell you this but Sophia was treated as my sister. It's impossible to understand what that little girl meant to me. Her laugh and her soulful eyes. Your daughter was, is and always will be a beautiful creature.

How will I manage without her? What will my working days look like when I can't see her smiling at me from the office door?

You know what a special person she is? Aura spoke and asked, her eyes filled with tears.

You shouldn't have been so upset. She was, is and will always be my daughter, as well as a good friend to those lucky enough to have known her. Your father replied, placing his hand on your shoulder.

Aaron placed ribbons of different colors with dedications on all windows in the house. Aaron wanted everyone to know how much he loved me. Next morning, everyone was tired, even those who hadn't slept, like Aaron's mother and father.

Aaron was wearing a black suit and I wore a long-curled wig. Unfortunately, I have yellow skin and closed eyes and Aaron's face is black and pale. As I drove to my final apartment, the sky began to fade and raindrops started falling on our car. It was a long road, but nobody felt alone. Every balcony from those in the building directly opposite Aaron's flat to the final station was decorated with ribbons.

The streets began to be filled with people and the rain seemed like it was cooling their faces.

People decide to get out of the car and go onto the balcony or the street. Red roses began to cover the street. Some fell from balconies and others from passing cars.

Alan, who was crying, played the piano right in the middle of town. I asked him to move and he did. He had to throw me a flower, so I stopped playing my violin. He kissed it and then threw the rose, saying aloud.

Alan - Fly beautiful angel, fly!

Henry never would have dressed up in a suit, especially not for me. Henry would only have been present at my joyous occasions. He didn't do much, apart from a few words with my dad. Aaron's workmates were very close because they all lacked experience in this situation.

Journalist: "Something extraordinary is happening right now. The whole city has been blocked off, and streets are filled up with red roses from balconies, as well as pedestrians who accompany the hearse. Sophia is the girl inside. Sophia was an inspiration to everyone, according to short interviews we were able to obtain from some people. It is believed that her death was caused by a lung condition.

Sophia donated her organs before she passed away. Her heart now beats in another person's body. Sophia is known for her amazing curly hair and smile throughout the city. Today, she shares a story.

The last greeting was filmed by the camera. Roses covered the ground in red and on every ribbon that was hung from balconies, it read:

Goodbye, SOPHIA

The words "On my cold and hard grave" were written.

Love is the mission of our lives!

The mission I set for myself was accomplished. I did what I could to give it another chance at life. And on the highest point of the city, there is a tree named Sophia.